ACSM's
Health-Related Physical Fitness
Assessment Manual
THIRD EDITION

>>

EDITOR

Leonard A. Kaminsky, PhD, FACSM
Coordinator, Clinical Exercise Physiology Program
Human Performance Laboratory
Ball State University
Muncie, Indiana

ACSM's
Health-Related
Physical Fitness
Assessment Manual

THIRD EDITION

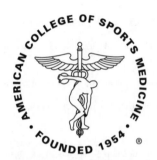

**AMERICAN COLLEGE
of SPORTS MEDICINE**®
w w w . a c s m . o r g

Wolters Kluwer | Lippincott Williams & Wilkins
Health

Philadelphia · Baltimore · New York · London
Buenos Aires · Hong Kong · Sydney · Tokyo

Acquisitions Editor: Emily Lupash
Managing Editor: Andrea Klingler
Marketing Manager: Christen Murphy
ACSM Group Publisher: Kerry O'Rourke
Compositor: Aptara, Inc

ACSM Committee on Certification and Registry Boards Chair: Dino Costanzo, MA, FACSM
ACSM Publications Committee Chair: Jeffrey L. Roitman, EdD, FACSM
ACSM Publications Committee Subchair: Janet P. Wallace, PhD, FACSM
ACSM Group Publisher: D. Mark Robertson, Assistant Executive Vice President

Third Edition

Printed in China

Library of Congress Cataloging-in-Publication Data

ACSM's health-related physical fitness assessment manual. — 3rd ed. / editor, Leonard Kaminsky ; American College of Sports Medicine.
          p. ; cm.
    Companion vol. to: ACSM's guidelines for exercise testing and prescription / American College of Sports Medicine. 8th ed. 2009.
    Includes bibliographical references and index.
    ISBN-13: 978-0-7817-9771-9
    ISBN-10: 0-7817-9771-3
  1. Physical fitness—Testing. 2. Exercise tests. I. Kaminsky, Leonard A., 1955– II. American College of Sports Medicine. III. American College of Sports Medicine. ACSM's guidelines for exercise testing and prescription. IV. Title: Health-related physical fitness assessment manual.
    [DNLM: 1. Physical Fitness—Guideline. 2. Exercise Test—standards—Guideline. 3. Physical Endurance—Guideline. 4. Physical Examination—standards—Guideline. QT 255 A187 2010]
    GV436.A35 2010
    613.7—dc22
                                                                                        2009008885

Care has been taken to confirm the accuracy of the information present and to describe generally accepted practices. However, the authors, editors, and publisher are not responsible for errors or omissions or for any consequences from application of the information in this book and make no warranty, expressed or implied, with respect to the currency, completeness, or accuracy of the contents of the publication. Application of this information in a particular situation remains the professional responsibility of the practitioner; the clinical treatments described and recommended may not be considered absolute and universal recommendations.

The authors, editors, and publisher have exerted every effort to ensure that drug selection and dosage set forth in this text are in accordance with the current recommendations and practice at the time of publication. However, in view of ongoing research, changes in government regulations, and the constant flow of information relating to drug therapy and drug reactions, the reader is urged to check the package insert for each drug for any change in indications and dosage and for added warnings and precautions. This is particularly important when the recommended agent is a new or infrequently employed drug.

Some drugs and medical devices presented in this publication have Food and Drug Administration (FDA) clearance for limited use in restricted research settings. It is the responsibility of the health care provider to ascertain the FDA status of each drug or device planned for use in their clinical practice.

To purchase additional copies of this book, call our customer service department at (800) 638-3030 or fax orders to (301) 223-2320. International customers should call (301) 223-2300.

Visit Lippincott Williams & Wilkins on the Internet: http://www.lww.com. Lippincott Williams & Wilkins customer service representatives are available from 8:30 am to 6:00 pm, EST.

For more information concerning American College of Sports Medicine certification and suggested preparatory materials, call (800) 486-5643 or visit the American College of Sports Medicine Website at www.acsm.org.

10 11 12 13
3 4 5 6 7 8 9

Preface

The American College of Sports Medicine has long been a leader in advocating the health benefits associated with a physical activity lifestyle. Recognition for the importance of performing regular physical activity for good health took a major leap forward with the release of the first-ever federal policy report, *Physical Activity Guidelines for Americans*, released in October 2008 by the U.S. Department of Health and Human Services (www.health.gov/PAguidelines/). Clinicians, public health professionals, and allied health professionals will now, more than ever, need the expertise of those trained and knowledgeable in prescribing physical activity/exercise and measuring the effects of these programs. As stated in Chapter 1 of this manual, physical fitness is the measurable outcome of a person's physical activity and exercise habits. Thus, it is essential that exercise professionals remain well versed in the methods of health-related physical fitness assessment and the interpretation of the results of these assessments.

This third edition of the ACSM's *Health-Related Physical Fitness Assessment Manual* updates the material from the previous editions and offers a significant amount of new material. The intent of this manual remains to provide a comprehensive overview of why and how to perform assessments of the five health-related components of physical fitness: body composition, muscular strength, muscular endurance, flexibility, and cardiorespiratory fitness. This manual is an extension of assessment principles covered in the ACSM's *Guidelines for Exercise Testing and Prescription* (8th edition) and includes many of the summary tables and figures from these *Guidelines*.

Readers familiar with the previous editions of this manual will notice the following new or significantly revised features in this third edition:

- New introductory material in Chapter 1 providing more background on issues related to health-related physical fitness.
- Reorganized and expanded information in Chapters 2 and 3 on preassessment screening and assessment of risk factors. These chapters include new material on blood sampling methods, assessment of physical activity, and assessment of risk of other chronic diseases, including pulmonary disease and osteoporosis.
- Reorganized material in Chapters 4–8 on the assessments of each of the components of health-related physical fitness. These chapters provide the background on the rationale for this assessment and the hierarchy of methods, with emphasis on the errors involved in prediction from lower-ordered methods. An overview of the major limitations of some assessment methods and a discussion of other unique assessment principles are provided.
- Step-by-step instructions for assessment of health-related physical fitness and resources for interpretation of test results. The manual provides more than 110 boxes, tables, and figures to help the reader understand the concepts of health-related physical fitness. There are a number of figures that demonstrate incorrect versus correct procedures of specific assessments.
- Case study analysis at the conclusion of each assessment chapter and suggested laboratories to help students master the concepts of health-related physical fitness.

Acknowledgments

When writing acknowledgments, one always runs the risk of omitting the mention of someone who has contributed. I am truly appreciative to all who provided support and assistance to the development of the third edition of this manual. With that being said, I do want to specifically acknowledge and thank the following individuals and groups.

Thanks to Dr. Greg Dwyer, who, through his teaching of fitness assessment to undergraduate Exercise Science students, recognized the need for a comprehensive manual of health-related physical fitness assessment. Greg, along with his coeditor, Dr. Shala Davis, produced the first two editions of this manual. All of us who teach, and the students who learn health-related physical fitness assessment, are indebted to you and Shala.

I appreciate all of the members of the American College of Sports Medicine who volunteer their time to our professional organization. I especially extend my gratitude to Dr. Jeff Pottinger and Dr. Jeff Roitman for asking me to serve as the editor of this third edition. I also wish to recognize Dr. Madeline Paternostro-Bayles and the team of reviewers for their timely work and contributions. Finally, thanks to the editorial groups of the eighth edition of *ACSM's Guidelines for Exercise Testing and Prescription* and the sixth edition of the *Resource Manual for the ACSM Guidelines for Exercise Testing and Prescription* for their cooperation throughout this project.

My gratitude to the professional staff of the American College of Sports Medicine who played an important role in this third edition, particularly Dr. Mark Robertson for the countless hours he served in the development of publications for this organization. I also want to recognize Kerry O'Rourke and Lori Tish for their support in the completion of this manual.

Thanks to the talented and hard-working staff at Lippincott Williams & Wilkins whom I have worked with now on three separate ACSM publications. I particularly want to extend my gratitude to Andrea Klingler and Matt Hauber for their assistance throughout this project.

Thanks to my professional colleagues who provided materials that contributed to this third edition: Dr. Tony Kaleth, Dr. Mark Kasper, Dr. Paul Nagelkirk, Mr. Jim Ross, Dr. Pat Schneider, Dr. Scott Strath, and Dr. Todd Trappe. I also extend my appreciation to my colleagues at Ball State University's Human Performance Laboratory, especially Lynn Clark, and to our graduate students for all of their support.

And finally, thank you to my wife, Mary, and my daughters, Lauren and Bonnie, for their continuing love and support. I also thank them for their behind-the-scenes assistance in support of the production of this manual.

Contents

Introduction

DEFINING HEALTH-RELATED PHYSICAL FITNESS

The purpose of *ACSM's Health-Related Physical Fitness Assessment Manual* is to provide a thorough overview of assessments of health-related physical fitness (HRPF). Physical fitness has been described in many different ways, as noted in Table 1.1, and thus, it is easy to get confused about the specific meaning of this common term. Brian Sharkey, PhD, professor emeritus of Montana State, notes, "Physical fitness is one of the most poorly defined and most frequently misused terms in the English Language."

Because it is important for allied health professionals to have a clear understanding of exactly what is meant by the term **physical fitness**, the Centers for Disease Control and Prevention (CDC) developed the following standard definition in 1985: ". . . a set of attributes or characteristics that people have or achieve that relates to the ability to perform physical activity" (2).

Health-related physical fitness, a more specific term, has been defined by the President's Council on Physical Fitness as consisting of those specific components of physical fitness that have a relationship with good health. Additionally, there are other components of physical fitness such as agility, balance, coordination, power, speed, and reaction time that are important for what is called sport- or skill-related physical fitness.

People achieve physical fitness through **exercise**, which the CDC defined as ". . . a type of physical activity consisting of planned, structured, and repetitive bodily movement done to improve or maintain one or more components of physical fitness."

The *ACSM's Guidelines for Exercise Testing and Prescription*, 8th edition (*GETP8*) provides specific guidelines for exercise training to improve HRPF (1).

Physical activity has been shown to be related to health and therefore is a term that must be clearly defined and understood. The CDC defined **physical activity** as "any bodily movement produced by the contraction of skeletal muscles that results in a substantial increase over resting energy expenditure."

It is important to use all the above terms correctly and have a clear understanding that physical fitness is a measurable set of characteristics that is determined by the exercise habits, or lack thereof, of an individual. Certainly, genetics also plays a role in the level of physical fitness one can achieve. Those with the highest levels of physical fitness have the optimal genetic makeup and have maximized their exercise training.

TABLE 1.1. DEFINITIONS OF PHYSICAL FITNESS

SOURCE	DEFINITION
Getchell (3)	Physical fitness is the capability of the heart, blood vessels, lungs, and muscles to perform at optimal efficiency.
Howley & Franks (5)	Fitness is the capacity to achieve the optimal quality of life.
Miller et al. (6)	General physical fitness is a state of ability to perform sustained physical work characterized by an effective integration of cardiorespiratory endurance, strength, flexibility, coordination, and body composition.
President's Council on Physical Fitness and Sports (8)	Physical fitness is the ability to carry out daily tasks with vigor and alertness without undue fatigue and ample energy to enjoy leisure-time pursuits and meet unforeseen emergencies.

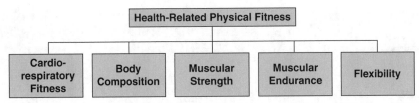

FIGURE 1.1. Health-related physical fitness is not a single entity, but rather a sum of five measurable components.

COMPONENTS OF HEALTH-RELATED PHYSICAL FITNESS

The American College of Sports Medicine (ACSM) has been a leader in setting guidelines for the assessment of physical fitness, particularly HRPF (1). There are five measurable components of HRPF as depicted in Figure 1.1.

3 *Cardiorespiratory endurance* refers to the ability of the circulatory and respiratory systems to supply oxygen during sustained physical activity. Cardiorespiratory fitness is related to the ability to perform large-muscle, dynamic, moderate- to high-intensity exercise for prolonged periods. The methods of assessment of cardiorespiratory fitness are provided in Chapters 7 and 8 of this manual.

Body composition refers to the relative amount or percentage of different types of body tissue (bone, fat, muscle) that are related to health. The most common health-related measure is that of total body fat percentage; however, it should be noted that there are no established criterion values for this measure related to health parameters. The methods used to assess body composition are provided in Chapter 4 of this manual.

Muscular strength is related to the ability to perform activities that require high levels of muscular force. Chapter 5 of this manual has specific measurement information on muscular strength.

Muscular endurance is the ability of a muscle group to execute repeated contractions over a period of time sufficient to cause muscular fatigue, or to maintain a specific percentage of the maximum voluntary contraction for a prolonged period of time. Chapter 5 of this manual has specific measurement information on muscular endurance.

Note: To better describe their integrated status, muscular strength and muscular endurance can be combined into one component of HRPF termed *muscular fitness*.

Flexibility is the ability to move a joint through its complete range of movement. Chapter 6 of this manual has specific measurement information on flexibility. Figure 1.2 displays one type of assessment of flexibility.

Even though an individual's appearance or exercise habits may be viewed as evidence of physical fitness and health, in reality, there is not one overall measure of physical fitness. Often regular exercisers spend most of their time training only one component of physical fitness. For example, the person who runs long distances 6 days per week may be considered "physically fit" (and indeed may be in terms of cardiorespiratory fitness); however, this person is often below average in terms of muscular strength and flexibility. Likewise, it is not uncommon for someone who performs high levels of resistance training as the sole form of exercise to be viewed as "physically fit" (and indeed may be in terms of muscular strength and muscular endurance); however, this person is often below average in terms of cardiorespiratory fitness and flexibility. Thus, it is important to view HRPF as an integration of the five components.

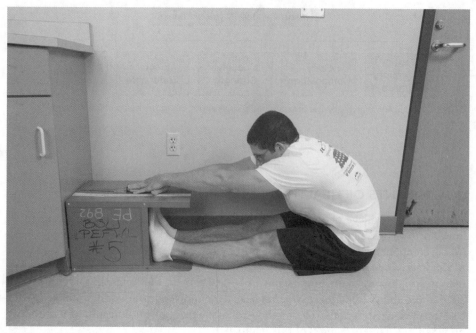

FIGURE 1.2. Flexibility is one of the components of health-related physical fitness.

THE IMPORTANCE OF MEASURING HEALTH-RELATED PHYSICAL FITNESS

THE RELATIONSHIP OF PHYSICAL FITNESS TO HEALTH

Scientific literature has firmly established the relationship between physical activity and health. Among the most notable publications asserting this relationship was the 1996 report from the U.S. Surgeon General entitled *Physical Activity and Health* (9). This report provided an extensive review of research demonstrating a variety of health-related benefits obtained from physical activity and also emphasized what is termed the *dose-response* relationship. The *dose* in this term refers to the amount of physical activity and/or exercise, whereas the *response* references the resultant health outcome. The evidence is quite clear that exercise doses do result in many health benefits as noted in Box 1.1. The exact minimal dose of physical activity and/or exercise that is required to produce health benefits is not yet clearly discerned; however, the ACSM and the American Heart Association have recently updated the recommendations for "Physical Activity and Public Health" (4). This publication is a must read for all exercise professionals. Remember that it is exercise that promotes the maintenance or improvement in physical fitness. In other words, physical fitness is the measurable outcome of a person's physical activity and exercise habits. Thus, the measurement of HRPF is becoming increasingly valued by many healthcare providers.

Among the important reasons for assessing HRPF, as cited in the *GETP8*, are the following:

- *Educating participants about their present health-related fitness status relative to health-related standards and age- and sex-matched norms.* Good healthcare for an individual

BOX 1.1   Benefits of Regular Physical Activity and/or Exercise

IMPROVEMENT IN CARDIOVASCULAR AND RESPIRATORY FUNCTION

- Increased maximal oxygen uptake owing to both central and peripheral adaptations
- Lower minute ventilation at a given submaximal intensity
- Lower myocardial oxygen cost for a given absolute submaximal intensity
- Lower heart rate and blood pressure at a given submaximal intensity
- Increased capillary density in skeletal muscle
- Increased exercise threshold for the accumulation of lactate in the blood
- Increased exercise threshold for the onset of disease signs or symptoms (e.g., angina pectoris, ischemic ST-segment depression, claudication)

REDUCTION IN CORONARY ARTERY DISEASE RISK FACTORS

- Reduced resting systolic/diastolic pressures
- Increased serum high-density lipoprotein cholesterol and decreased serum triglycerides
- Reduced total body fat, reduced intra-abdominal fat
- Reduced insulin needs, improved glucose tolerance

DECREASED MORTALITY AND MORBIDITY

- Primary prevention (i.e., interventions to prevent an acute cardiac event)
  - Higher activity and/or fitness levels are associated with lower death rates from coronary artery disease
  - Higher activity and/or fitness levels are associated with lower incidence rates for combined cardiovascular diseases, coronary artery disease, cancer of the colon, and type 2 diabetes
- Secondary prevention (i.e., interventions after a cardiac event [to prevent another])
  - Based on meta-analyses (pooled data across studies), cardiovascular and all-cause mortality are reduced in postmyocardial infarction patients who participate in cardiac rehabilitation exercise training, especially as a component of multifactorial risk factor reduction[a]

OTHER POSTULATED BENEFITS

- Decreased anxiety and depression
- Enhanced physical function and independent living in older persons
- Enhanced feelings of well-being
- Enhanced performance of work, recreational, and sport activities
- Reduced risk of falls and injuries from falls in older persons
- Prevention or mitigation of functional limitations in older persons
- Effective therapy for many chronic diseases in older adults

[a]Randomized controlled trials of cardiac rehabilitation exercise training involving postmyocardial infarction patients do not support a reduction in the rate of nonfatal reinfarction

Adapted from American College of Sports Medicine. *ACSM's Guidelines for Exercise Testing and Prescription*, 8th ed. Philadelphia (PA): Wolters Kluwer Health Ltd: 2009, 9–10 p.

includes knowing important personal health-related information such as one's cholesterol level and blood pressure. Similarly, knowledge of HRPF measurements would support optimizing personal health.

- *Providing data that are helpful in the development of exercise prescriptions to address all fitness components.* Maintenance or improvement in the different components of HRPF requires different types of exercise training. Thus, although there are some generalized exercise recommendations for good health, the exercise prescription can and should be tailored to the specific needs and goals of the individual. This is best achieved by having current HRPF measurements.
- *Collecting baseline and follow-up data that allow evaluation of progress by exercise program participants.* Other personal health information, such as cholesterol and blood pressure, is tracked over time. Similarly, measuring HRPF periodically can aid an individual in managing personal health. Measurements through time can also help identify whether the training program needs to be modified to improve some components of HRPF while maintaining desired levels of the other components of HRPF.
- *Motivating participants by establishing reasonable and attainable fitness goals.* Knowing one's HRPF measures provides a basis for individualizing a physical fitness program. Periodic assessments allow tracking progress toward meeting goals.
- *Stratifying cardiovascular risk.* Two of the components of HRPF, cardiorespiratory fitness and body composition, are directly related to cardiovascular disease risk. More information on risk factor assessment and determining a risk stratification classification is provided in Chapters 2 and 3.

THE RELATIONSHIP OF PHYSICAL FITNESS TO FUNCTION

It has been well recognized that many aspects of sport performance are related to physical fitness. Indeed, there are several sport-related physical fitness components such as power, agility, and balance that can be assessed. Although not necessarily related to a specific performance outcome, the components of HRPF are now being recognized as important to the function of everyday tasks and leisure-time pursuits. For example, consider a household task such as a landscaping project at home that will require lifting bags that could weigh between 10 and 50 pounds, repeatedly shoveling materials into a wheelbarrow, and bending and reaching. These tasks require sufficient levels of muscular strength, muscular endurance, and flexibility. Also, consider the opportunity to accept an invitation to travel with a group that will be taking a camping trip to a scenic wilderness location. This experience will involve a fair degree of hiking and the ability to perform this activity will require a certain level of cardiorespiratory fitness and muscular endurance and will be influenced by body composition.

These are only two examples of how HRPF is related to function. Certainly the performance of many of the activities of daily living depends on one's physical fitness level, and this becomes even more apparent as one ages. Figure 1.3 shows an example of a recreational activity that can be performed throughout one's lifetime if one maintains an adequate level of HRPF.

FUNDAMENTAL PRINCIPLES OF ASSESSMENT

For each of the components of HRPF, there are a variety of assessment methods that can be used. Chapters 4–8 of this manual will provide an overview of assessment procedures

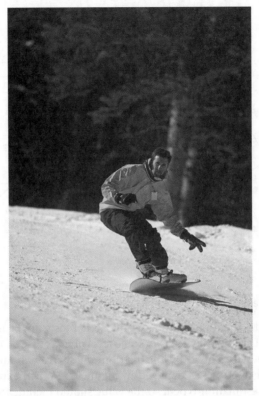

FIGURE 1.3. People who are physically fit are capable of performing both occupational and recreational activities throughout their lifetimes.

and interpretations for each of the components of HRPF. However, regardless of which component of HRPF is assessed, there are fundamental principles that should be applied in performing physical fitness assessments.

A SPECIFIC ASSESSMENT OBJECTIVE

There should be a clear purpose identified prior to performing the assessment. A list of important reasons for performing HRPF measurements is provided on the previous page. It is important for both the client and the physical fitness professional to have an understanding of what the objective is for the assessment. Knowing the objective of the assessment will ensure the selection of the most appropriate procedure.

THE GOLD STANDARD (i.e., TRUE MEASURE)

A general principle in assessment is that one test is considered the criterion test or gold standard; that is, it is considered the definitive or true measure. This does not necessarily mean that it is a perfect test, but that it is considered the best test that exists for measuring a specific variable. Although ideal, the gold standard test may not always be utilized owing to several different circumstances such as the need for expensive equipment and trained personnel, the requirement of extensive time, and the increased risks involved.

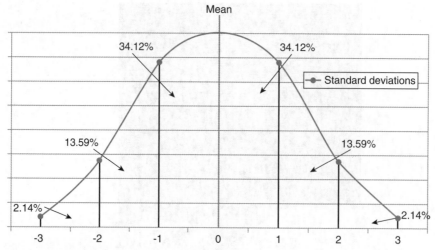

FIGURE 1.4. The characteristics of the normal bell curve.

Error of Measurement

If the use of the gold standard test is not feasible, other tests can be used to estimate the variable of interest. This typically leads to some level of inaccuracy. For most physiologic variables, such as measures of HRPF, the distribution of errors in measurement follows that of the normal bell curve, as depicted in Figure 1.4. When expressing a measurement value from an estimation-type test, the value should include the error range. This is typically expressed as ±1 standard deviation from the mean, or in prediction equations the standard error of estimate (SEE). Say, for example, the test used reported a value of 50 ± 5. This means that if there were 100 cases with a value estimated to be 50, 68 of those cases would have an actual value between 45 and 55, 95 of the cases would have an actual value between 40 and 60, and five cases would have values either <40 or >60. Specifics about measurement errors for different HRPF tests will be provided in Chapters 4–8. Thus, it is important for the physical fitness professional to understand the amount of error in measurement when utilizing indirect tests to estimate an HRPF component.

EQUIPMENT CALIBRATION

Some instruments or equipment used provide accurate measurements every time if used correctly. For example, a wall-mounted stadiometer is a stable device that measures distance accurately. However, a device such as a weight scale may over time produce different readings for standard weight. To ensure the accuracy of the reading, the device must be calibrated prior to the testing session and properly adjusted to produce an accurate reading.

STANDARDIZATION

Another important fundamental for assessment is following standardized procedures. Many factors can cause variability in a measurement, so uniform standards need to be applied to reduce or eliminate the sources of variability. These may include pretest instructions that may extend to the time 24 hours prior to the test (e.g., no vigorous exercise on the day prior to the test) and the environmental conditions of the fitness testing facility (e.g., temperature between 20°C and 24°C).

INTERPRETATION ISSUES

Ideally there exists one standard that can be used to interpret the results of a test. For example, it is well accepted that in a health assessment that includes a total cholesterol measurement, the results are interpreted with the values established by the National Cholesterol Education Program (NCEP) (7). Unfortunately, no national set of standards has been established for HRPF assessment interpretation.

Types of Standards

There are two basic types of standards: criterion-referenced and normative. Criterion-referenced standards are a set of scores that classify the result as desirable (or above or below desirable) based on some external criteria, such as the betterment of health (a group of experts has determined what is desirable). Criterion-referenced standards often thus use adjectives such as "excellent" or "poor" in classifying test results. Normative standards, sometimes referred to as norms, are based on the past performance of groups of individuals with similar characteristics (e.g., age, gender). Thus, with normative standards, a comparison is made between the client's performance and the performance of similar individuals. The data interpretation classifications often use a percentile score, such as 90th, 50th, etc. In HRPF assessment, there are more normative standards than criterion-referenced standards available for interpretation.

THE PHYSICAL FITNESS PROFESSIONAL

Webster defines a professional as one who "conforms to the technical and ethical standards of his or her profession." A profession is "a calling requiring specialized knowledge and often long and intensive academic preparation."

There are no defined professional standards for those who work with people in the areas of physical fitness or exercise. However, some states have pursued licensure legislation that would set standards for professionals that provide these services. Additionally, some employers have voluntarily set standards for individuals they hire to perform physical fitness assessments or to supervise exercise programs.

ACADEMIC TRAINING

For many years, universities have offered degrees focused on exercise, many of these originating out of Physical Education programs. The exact title of the degree (e.g., Exercise Physiology, Exercise Science, Kinesiology) is unique to the institution, as is the required curriculum. Degrees are offered at the associate, bachelor's, master's, and doctoral levels. Some professional organizations, including ACSM, have initiated efforts to support accreditation of academic programs that offer degree programs in Exercise Science.

CREDENTIALS

Many people who work in the area of physical fitness assessment and/or in providing exercise program services obtain a certification, usually from a professional organization, that attests they have achieved a minimal level of knowledge and/or competency. Although there are literally hundreds of different organizations and groups that offer some form of certification related to physical fitness assessment and/or exercise services, ACSM has been a leader in providing these types of certifications. Presently ACSM offers four different types of certifications, with prerequisite requirements ranging from being 18 years old with a high school degree (ACSM Certified Personal Trainer[SM]) to having a master's degree in Exercise Science with a minimum of 600 hours of clinical work experience (ACSM Registered Clinical Exercise Physiologist[®]). Appendix D of the *GETP8* provides detailed information about these ACSM certifications.

REFERENCES

1. American College of Sports Medicine. *Guidelines for Exercise Testing and Prescription.* 8th ed. Philadelphia: 2009 Lippincott Williams & Wilkins.
2. Caspersen CJ, Powell KE, Christenson GM. Physical activity, exercise, and physical fitness: definitions and distinctions for health-related research. *Public Health Rep.* 1985;100(2):126–31.
3. Getchell B. *Physical Fitness: A Way of Life.* New York: 1992 Macmillian Publishing Co. 8 p.
4. Haskell WL, Lee IM, Pate RR, et al. Physical activity and public health: updated recommendation from the American College of Sports Medicine and the American Heart Association. *Med Sci Sports Exerc.* 2007;39: 1423–43.
5. Howley ET, Franks BD. *Health/Fitness Instructor's Handbook.* Champaign (IL): 1986 Human Kinetics. 4 p.
6. Miller AJ, Grais IM, Winslow E, Kaminsky LA. The definition of physical fitness. *J Sports Med Phys Fitness.* 1991;31:639–40.
7. National Cholesterol Education Program. *Third Report of the National Cholesterol Education Program (NCEP) Expert Panel on Detection, Evaluation, and Treatment of High Blood Cholesterol in Adults (Adult Treatment Panel III).* Washington, DC: 2002 NIH Publication No. 02-5215.
8. President's Council on Physical Fitness and Sports. *Physical Fitness Research Digest.* Washington, DC: 1971 President's Council on Physical Fitness and Sports.
9. U.S. Department of Health and Human Services and Centers for Disease Control and Prevention. *Physical Activity and Health: A Report of the Surgeon General.* Atlanta (GA): 1996 National Center for Chronic Disease Prevention and Health Promotion.

Preassessment Screening

RATIONALE FOR PREASSESSMENT SCREENING

Most of the health-related physical fitness (HRPF) assessment procedures involve performing exercise, and in some cases the level of exertion required is vigorous to maximal. Risks of both cardiovascular and musculoskeletal injuries are associated with exercise. These risks increase with the intensity of the exercise, as indicated in this statement from *ACSM's Guidelines for Exercise Testing and Prescription*, 8th edition (*GETP8*): "There is an acute and transient increase in the risk of sudden cardiac death and/or myocardial infarction in individuals performing vigorous exercise with either diagnosed or occult cardiovascular disease."

More specific information about cardiovascular risks associated with exercise resides in Chapter 1 of the *GETP8*, with summarized data about event rates found in that text's Tables 1.4, 1.5, and 1.6.

Similarly, the risks for musculoskeletal injuries are greater in those individuals with known musculoskeletal diseases or previous injuries and those who are inactive. Therefore, it is critical to know the health status and history of all individuals who will be performing HRPF assessments.

The first contact most individuals have with a program is with the person who administers the informed consent and conducts the risk stratification screening. The client's impression of a program may depend on this first contact with the staff. Thinking about fitness testing may create anxiety in the client and the test results may create other feelings that are not pleasurable. Every effort should be made to help the client relax and focus on the beneficial information afforded from the results of the HRPF assessment. Although the exact approach may vary somewhat depending on the client's personality, performing this initial stage of the assessment with calm professionalism is recommended.

INFORMED CONSENT

The first step in the process of HRPF assessment is completion of the informed consent. This step must precede the health risk appraisal because determination of the health risk status will require the exchange of private health information and may require procedures that involve physical risk (e.g., blood testing).

The essential steps in executing the informed consent are:

- Explaining the purpose of the assessments
- Describing the procedures to be used
- Describing the risks and discomforts associated with the assessments
- Describing the benefits obtained from the assessments
- Describing alternatives (if any)
- Describing the responsibilities required of the client
- Encouraging the client to ask questions at any time
- Explaining how data will be handled (confidentiality)
- Explaining that the client can withdraw his or her consent and stop the assessment process at any time

An example of an informed consent form is provided in Box 2.1. It is important to note, however, that there are many variations of informed consent forms available from different sources. All professionals performing assessments should take the time to find a standard form that closely matches their facility's needs and assessments.

BOX 2.1 | **An Example of an Informed Consent Document for Health-Related Physical Fitness (HRPF) Assessment**

1. Purpose and explanation of the test
   This test will provide an estimation of your cardiorespiratory fitness. You will perform a submaximal exercise test on a cycle ergometer. The exercise intensity will begin at a low level and will be advanced in stages depending on your fitness level. We may stop the test at any time because of signs of fatigue or changes in your heart rate or blood pressure, or symptoms you may experience. It is important for you to realize that you may stop when you wish because of feelings of fatigue or any other discomfort.

2. Attendant risks and discomforts
   There exists the possibility of certain changes occurring during the test. These include abnormal blood pressure; fainting; irregular, fast, or slow heart rhythm; and, in rare instances, heart attack, stroke, or death. Every effort will be made to minimize these risks by evaluation of preliminary information relating to your health and fitness and by careful observations during testing. Emergency equipment and trained personnel are available to deal with unusual situations that may arise.

3. Responsibilities of the participant
   Information you possess about your health status or previous experiences of heart-related symptoms (e.g., shortness of breath with low-level activity, pain, pressure, tightness, heaviness in the chest, neck, jaw, back, and/or arms) with physical effort may affect the safety of your exercise test. Your prompt reporting of these and any other unusual feelings with effort during the exercise test itself is very important. You are responsible for fully disclosing your medical history, as well as symptoms that may occur during the test. You are also expected to report all medications (including nonprescription) taken recently and, in particular, those taken today to the testing staff.

4. Benefits to be expected
   The results obtained from the exercise test may assist in the development of an individualized exercise prescription and will provide information that will be helpful in tracking your potential cardiorespiratory fitness changes over time.

5. Inquiries
   Any questions about the procedures used in the exercise test or the results of your test are encouraged. If you have any concerns or questions, please ask us for further explanations.

6. Use of medical records
   The information that is obtained during exercise testing will be treated as privileged and confidential as described in the Health Insurance Portability and Accountability Act of 1996. It is not to be released or revealed to any person except your referring physician without your written consent. However, the information obtained may be used for statistical analysis or scientific purposes with your right to privacy retained.

Box 2.1. continued

---

7. Freedom of consent

I hereby consent to voluntarily engage in an exercise test to estimate my cardiorespiratory fitness. My permission to perform this exercise test is given voluntarily. I understand that I am free to stop the test at any point if I so desire.

I have read this form, and I understand the test procedures that I will perform and the attendant risks and discomforts. Knowing these risks and discomforts, and having had an opportunity to ask questions that have been answered to my satisfaction, I consent to participate in this test.

_____   _____

Date   Signature of Client

_____   _____

Date   Signature of Witness

Adapted from American College of Sports Medicine. *ACSM's Guidelines for Exercise Testing and Prescription*, 8th ed. Philadelphia (PA): Wolters Kluwer Health Ltd: 2009, 56–57 p. Figure 3-1.

Modifications to the form can be made to fit specific needs of the HRPF assessment program, and it is recommended that legal counsel review the final form to limit the chances of legal liability. Finally, it is essential that different informed consent forms be used for each different component of a program (i.e., assessments and exercise programs).

THE PROCESS OF THE INFORMED CONSENT

It is important to understand that the informed consent is not just a form requiring a signature. Rather, it is a process of documentation that attests to the fact that clear communications have taken place between the individual who is desiring to have the HRPF assessment and the professional who will be administering the assessments. It is through the process of articulating the risks and benefits of the assessment that professionals help their clients make informed decisions about whether to complete the HRPF assessment. Although the evidence suggests that for most people expected benefits of performing the assessment outweigh the associated risks, each client needs to make an informed decision based on personal factors.

To begin the informed consent process, the client should carefully read the entire form or have the form read to him or her while he or she follows along. Next, the professional should review some of the key elements of the assessment (e.g., purpose, risks and benefits, overview of procedures; Fig. 2.1). One key point of emphasis is that the client will play an important role in the process. Specifically, the client has the responsibility of informing test administrators of any problems experienced (past, present, and during the physical fitness assessment) that may increase the risk of the test or preclude participation. This information is essential to minimize the risks involved with the assessment and can optimize the benefits. Finally, the client should be allowed and encouraged to ask any questions before completing the informed consent process with a signature.

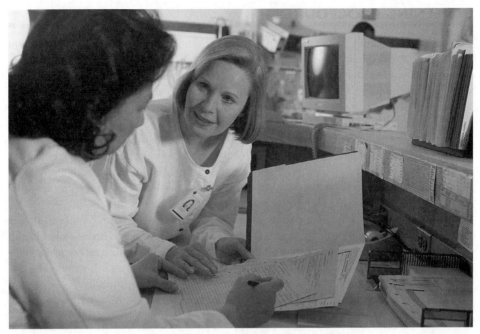

FIGURE 2.1. An important aspect of the informed consent process is reviewing key elements with the client and answering any questions the client may have.

EXPLANATION OF PROCEDURES

The professional should be prepared to provide a brief description of each assessment to be performed and answer client questions in detail. Below are examples of some common HRPF assessments and sample explanations of each. More detailed review of all the HRPF assessments is covered in Chapters 4–8.

- Anthropometry or body composition: "This test is being performed to obtain an estimate of your total body fat percentage. We will determine your body fat percentage by taking measurements with a set of calipers at different sites on your body. We do this by pinching and pulling on the skin at these different locations. We will also measure some body girths with a tape measure to provide an indication of distribution of the fat on your body."
- Cardiorespiratory fitness: "This test is being performed to obtain an estimate of your cardiorespiratory fitness. The test will require you to exercise on a stationary cycle for 6 to 12 minutes. The intensity of the test will be limited to a level below your maximal exertion point. During the test we will monitor your heart rate and blood pressure response to the submaximal exercise."
- Flexibility: "This test is being performed to obtain a measure of the flexibility of your lower back and legs. We will measure how far you can reach to or beyond your toes while sitting with your knees out straight."
- Muscular fitness: "This test is being performed to obtain a measure of your muscle strength by having you squeeze a hand grip dynamometer as hard as you can. We will also measure muscle endurance by having you perform as many sit-ups as you can in a 1-minute time period."

SCREENING PROCEDURES

Preassessment screening is the next step in the process of HRPF assessment. Preassessment screening is a process of gathering a client's demographic and health-related information, along with some health risk/medical assessments (see Chapter 3). This information may be used for determining the individual's risks for chronic disease and risks related to physical activity participation. As noted earlier in this chapter, there are risks associated with exercise, particularly when it is of vigorous intensity. As reviewed in the *GETP8*, because of these risks, the U.S. Surgeon General in the 1996 Report on Physical Activity and Health (3) recommended that "Previously inactive men over age 40, women over age 50, and people at high risk for CVD [cardiovascular disease] should first consult a physician before embarking on a program of vigorous physical activity to which they are unaccustomed. People with disease should be evaluated by a physician first...."

The preassessment screening, like the informed consent, is a dynamic process. It may vary in its scope and components depending on the client's needs based on his or her health and medical status (e.g., health conditions or diseases), the type of HRPF assessments gathered (e.g., submaximal vs. maximal cardiorespiratory fitness tests), and the physical activity or exercise program goals (e.g., moderate intensity vs. vigorous intensity).

There are many reasons why clients should be screened prior to participation in an HRPF assessment program. These include:

- To identify those with a medical contraindication (exclusion), as outlined in Box 2.2, to performing specific HRPF assessments
- To identify those who should receive a medical evaluation conducted by a physician prior to performing specific HRPF assessments
- To identify those who should only perform HRPF assessments administered by professionals with clinical experience (and possibly in a clinical facility with physician availability)
- To identify those with other health risk/medical concerns (e.g., diabetes mellitus or orthopedic injuries) that may influence the decision about performing specific HRPF assessments or the need to modify assessment procedures

OBJECTIVE: RISK STRATIFICATION

To stratify is to divide or separate into levels or classes, called strata. The *GETP8* has a specific set of guidelines for preactivity screening and supervision requirements for exercise tests (fitness assessments) based on the client's level of risk. The purpose of risk stratification is to help determine the appropriate course of action regarding fitness assessments involving exercise testing. This should be done as a screening for an individual planning on beginning an exercise program. There are three risk stratification classifications developed for individuals for this purpose as defined in Table 2.1.

Figure 2.2 provides an example of the logic involved in this decision-making process. Specifically, the first decision must determine whether a medical examination is recommended prior to the HRPF assessment. If a medical exam is not deemed necessary, then the next decision determines the appropriate level of the assessment (usually related to the intensity of exercise) and whether any assessments should be performed with clinical supervision. Always remember, however, that this stratification process is only a recommended guide for action. Fitness professionals should always use prudent judgment when deciding whether a client needs a physician's clearance prior to HRPF assessment. If unsure, select the conservative option and require a physician's clearance.

BOX 2.2	**Contraindications for Exercise Testing**

ABSOLUTE

- A recent significant change in the resting ECG suggesting significant ischemia, recent myocardial infarction (within 2 days), or other acute cardiac event
- Unstable angina
- Uncontrolled cardiac dysrhythmias causing symptoms or hemodynamic compromise
- Symptomatic severe aortic stenosis
- Uncontrolled symptomatic heart failure
- Acute pulmonary embolus or pulmonary infarction
- Acute myocarditis or pericarditis
- Suspected or known dissecting aneurysm
- Acute systemic infection, accompanied by fever, body aches, or swollen lymph glands

RELATIVE[a]

- Left main coronary stenosis
- Moderate stenotic valvular heart disease
- Electrolyte abnormalities (e.g., hypokalemia, hypomagnesemia)
- Severe arterial hypertension (i.e., systolic BP of >200 mmHg and/or a diastolic BP of >110 mmHg) at rest
- Tachydysrhythmia or bradydysrhythmia
- Hypertrophic cardiomyopathy and other forms of outflow tract obstruction
- Neuromuscular, musculoskeletal, or rheumatoid disorders that are exacerbated by exercise
- High-degree atrioventricular block
- Ventricular aneurysm
- Uncontrolled metabolic disease (e.g., diabetes, thyrotoxicosis, or myxedema)
- Chronic infectious disease (e.g., mononucleosis, hepatitis, AIDS)
- Mental or physical impairment leading to inability to exercise adequately

[a]Relative contraindications can be superseded if benefits outweigh risks of exercise. In some instances, these individuals can be exercised with caution and/or using low-level end points, especially if they are asymptomatic at rest.

Adapted from American College of Sports Medicine. *ACSM's Guidelines for Exercise Testing and Prescription,* 8th ed. Philadelphia (PA): Wolters Kluwer Health Ltd: 2009, 54 p.

Modified from Gibbons RJ, Balady GJ, Bricker J, et al. ACC/AHA 2002 guideline update for exercise testing: a report of the American College of Cardiology/American Heart Association Task Force on Practice Guidelines (Committee on Exercise Testing). *Circulation*:106(14);1883–1892, with permission.

HEALTH HISTORY QUESTIONNAIRE

Most of the pertinent health risks and medical information about a client can be obtained from a health history questionnaire (HHQ). The HHQ, along with results from risk assessments, determines the client's risk stratification level. The HHQ can be tailored to fit the specific information required of the type of HRPF assessment being performed. For example, little health risk and medical information is needed if the

TABLE 2.1. ACSM RISK STRATIFICATION CATEGORIES FOR ATHEROSCLEROTIC CARDIOVASCULAR DISEASE (CVD)

Low risk	Asymptomatic men and women who have ≤1 CVD risk factor from Table 2.2
Moderate risk	Asymptomatic men and women who have ≥2 risk factors from Table 2.2
High risk	Individuals who have known cardiovascular,[a] pulmonary,[b] or metabolic[c] disease or ≥ signs and symptoms listed in Table 2.3

ACSM, American College of Sports Medicine; CVD, cardiovascular disease.

[a]Cardiac, peripheral vascular, or cerebrovascular disease.

[b]Chronic obstructive pulmonary disease, asthma, interstitial lung disease, or cystic fibrosis.

[c]Diabetes mellitus (type 1, type 2), thyroid disorders, renal, or liver disease.

Adapted from American College of Sports Medicine. *ACSM's Guidelines for Exercise Testing and Prescription,* 8th ed. Philadelphia (PA): Wolters Kluwer Health Ltd: 2009, 23 p.

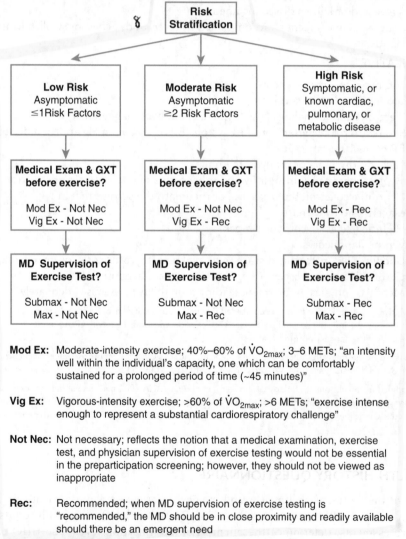

Mod Ex: Moderate-intensity exercise; 40%–60% of $\dot{V}O_{2max}$; 3–6 METs; "an intensity well within the individual's capacity, one which can be comfortably sustained for a prolonged period of time (~45 minutes)"

Vig Ex: Vigorous-intensity exercise; >60% of $\dot{V}O_{2max}$; >6 METs; "exercise intense enough to represent a substantial cardiorespiratory challenge"

Not Nec: Not necessary; reflects the notion that a medical examination, exercise test, and physician supervision of exercise testing would not be essential in the preparticipation screening; however, they should not be viewed as inappropriate

Rec: Recommended; when MD supervision of exercise testing is "recommended," the MD should be in close proximity and readily available should there be an emergent need

FIGURE 2.2. Exercise testing and testing supervision recommendations based on risk stratification. GXT, graded exercise test; METs, metabolic equivalents. (From American College of Sports Medicine. *ACSM's Guidelines for Exercise Testing and Prescription,* 8th ed. Philadelphia [PA]: Wolters Kluwer Health Ltd: 2009, 32 p.)

client is only performing a body composition assessment. However, clients interested in performing assessments requiring maximal exercise should complete a comprehensive HHQ. In general, the HHQ should assess a client's:

- Cardiovascular disease risk factors
- Past history of any signs and symptoms suggestive of cardiovascular disease
- Personal history of chronic diseases and illnesses
- History of surgeries and hospitalizations
- History of any musculoskeletal and joint injuries
- Past and present health behaviors/habits (physical activity, dietary patterns, weight loss)
- Current use of any medications

An example of a comprehensive health history form is shown in Figure 2.3.

Cardiovascular Disease Risk Factors

The cardiovascular disease risk factors' thresholds used in the American College of Sports Medicine (ACSM) risk stratification process are listed in Table 2.2. To determine levels of risk, the ACSM uses criteria established by other professional organizations such as the National Cholesterol Education Program (NCEP). However, slightly different risk factor criteria may be found in some other sources. Remember that the risk stratification classification is used to make decisions regarding the recommendation for a medical exam prior to participating in an HRPF assessment and for the types of testing and supervision recommended.

It is important to follow the specific criteria for determining the presence or absence of the cardiovascular disease risk factors. For example, note that age thresholds differ between the age risk factor and the family history risk factor. Also, for the blood pressure and hyperlipidemia risk factors, repeat assessments are necessary to confirm the measurement, and those whose conditions are controlled by medications are still considered to have the risk factors.

The risk stratification classification of a client is determined by the numerical total of all risk factors. Note that there are eight positive risk factors and one negative risk factor used by ACSM for risk stratification. If a client has high high-density lipoprotein (HDL) cholesterol, then 1 is subtracted from the sum of the positive risk factors to determine the total number of risk factors for risk stratification.

Signs or Symptoms Suggestive of Cardiopulmonary Disease

There are several visible signs or reported symptoms a client may have that would indicate the likelihood of having a cardiovascular, pulmonary, or metabolic disease. These signs and symptoms are listed in Table 2.3. If a client has any of these signs or symptoms, then the client is placed in the high-risk stratification classification, regardless of the presence or absence of any cardiovascular disease risk factors. A client with a sign or symptom should be immediately referred to a physician for follow-up.

To make a decision about the presence or absence of a sign or symptom suggestive of cardiovascular, pulmonary, or metabolic disease, be sure to follow the specific criteria. Some key features that aid in clarifying whether the reported feeling should be designated as a symptom are listed in Table 2.3. For example, a client may report that he/she

TODAY'S DATE _____

NAME _____ AGE _____   DATE OF BIRTH _____

ADDRESS _____
              Street   City   State   Zip

TELEPHONE: HOME/CELL _____/ _____E-MAIL ADDRESS _____

OCCUPATION/EMPLOYER _____/ _____ BUSINESS PHONE _____

MARITAL STATUS: (check one) SINGLE ☐   MARRIED ☐   DIVORCED ☐   WIDOWED ☐

PERSONAL PHYSICIAN _____ PHONE # _____

ADDRESS _____

Reason for last doctor visit?_____ Date of last physical exam: _____

Have you ever had any other exercise stress test?   YES ☐   NO ☐   DATE & LOCATION OF TEST: _____
_____

Have you ever had any cardiovascular tests?   YES ☐   NO ☐   DATE & LOCATION: _____
_____

Person to contact in case of an emergency _____ Phone _____ (relationship) _____

Please provide responses (YES or NO) to the following concerning family history, your own history, and any symptoms you have had:

FAMILY HISTORY		
Have any immediate family members had a:		
	YES	NO
heart attack	o	o
heart surgery	o	o
coronary stent	o	o
cardiac catheterization	o	o
congenital heart defect	o	o
stroke	o	o
Other chronic disease: _____		
_____		
_____		
_____		
_____		

PERSONAL HISTORY		
Have you ever had:		
	YES	NO
High blood pressure	o	o
High cholesterol	o	o
Diabetes	o	o
Any heart problems	o	o
Disease of arteries	o	o
Thyroid disease	o	o
Lung disease	o	o
Asthma	o	o
Cancer	o	o
Kidney disease	o	o
Hepatitis	o	o
Other: _____		
_____		

SYMPTOMS		
Have you ever had:		
	YES	NO
Chest pain	o	o
Shortness of breath	o	o
Heart palpitations	o	o
Skipped heartbeats	o	o
Heart murmur	o	o
Intermittent leg pain	o	o
Dizziness or fainting	o	o
Fatigue — usual activities	o	o
Snoring	o	o
Back pain	o	o
Orthopedic problems	o	o
Other: _____		
_____		

STAFF COMMENTS: _____
_____
_____

Have you ever had your cholesterol measured?   Yes ☐   No ☐   If yes, value _____ Where: _____

Are you taking any prescription (include birth control pills) or nonprescription medications?   Yes ☐   No ☐
For each of your current medications, provide the following information:

MEDICATION   Dosage—times/day   Time taken   Years on medication   Reason for taking

_____
_____
_____

FIGURE 2.3. An example of a comprehensive health history questionnaire (HHQ). (Source: Ball State University – Clinical Exercise Physiology Program.)

HOSPITALIZATIONS: Please list recent hospitalizations (Women: do not list normal pregnancies)

Year   Location   Reason

_____

_____

_____

Any other medical problems/concerns not already identified?   Yes ☐   No ☐   If so, please list: _____

_____

_____

LIFESTYLE HABITS

Do you ever have an uncomfortable shortness of breath during exercise or when doing activities?
   Yes ☐   No ☐

Do you ever have chest discomfort during exercise?   Yes ☐   No ☐
   If so, does it go away with rest?   Yes ☐   No ☐

_____

Do you currently smoke?   Yes ☐   No ☐   If so, what? Cigarettes ☐   Cigars ☐   Pipe ☐
   How long have you smoked? _____ years

How much per day: <½ pack ☐   ½ to 1 pack ☐   1 to 1½ packs ☐   1½ to 2 packs ☐   >2 packs ☐

Have you ever quit smoking?   Yes ☐   No ☐   When? _____
   How many years and how much did you smoke? _____

Do you drink any alcoholic beverages?   Yes ☐   No ☐   If yes, how much in 1 week? (indicate below)
   Beer _____ (cans)   Wine _____ (glasses)   Hard liquor _____ (drinks)

Do you drink any caffeinated beverages?   Yes ☐   No ☐   If yes, how much in 1 week? (indicate below)
   Coffee _____ (cups)   Tea _____ (glasses)   Soft drinks _____ (cans)

Are you currently following a weight reduction diet plan?   Yes ☐   No ☐
   If so, how long have you been dieting? _____ months
   Is the plan prescribed by your doctor?   Yes ☐   No ☐

Have you used weight reduction diets in the past?   Yes ☐   No ☐   If yes, how often and what type? _____

_____

ACTIVITY LEVEL EVALUATION

What is your occupational activity level?   Sedentary ☐   Light ☐   Moderate ☐   Heavy ☐

Do you currently engage in vigorous physical activity on a regular basis?   Yes ☐   No ☐
   If so, what type(s)? _____ How many days per week? _____
   How much time per day?   <15 min ☐   15-30 min ☐   31-60 min ☐   >60 min ☐
   How long have you engaged in this type of activity?   <3 months ☐   3-12 months ☐   >1 year ☐

_____

Do you engage in any recreational or leisure-time physical activities on a regular basis?   Yes ☐   No ☐
   If so, what activities? _____
   On average: How often? _____ times/week;   for how long? _____ time/session
   How long have you engaged in this type of activity?   <3 months   3-12 months   >1 year

_____

Your fitness goals and objectives are: _____

_____

STAFF COMMENTS: _____

_____

_____

FIGURE 2.3. *Continued.*

TABLE 2.2. ATHEROSCLEROTIC CARDIOVASCULAR DISEASE (CVD) RISK FACTOR THRESHOLDS FOR USE WITH ACSM RISK STRATIFICATION

POSITIVE RISK FACTORS	DEFINING CRITERIA
Age	Men ≥45 yr; Women ≥55 yr
Family history	Myocardial infarction, coronary revascularization, or sudden death before 55 yr of age in father or other male first-degree relative, or before 65 yr of age in mother or other female first-degree relative
Cigarette smoking	Current cigarette smoker or those who quit within the previous 6 months or exposure to environmental tobacco smoke
Sedentary lifestyle	Not participating in at least 30 min of moderate intensity (40%–60% $\dot{V}O_2R$) physical activity on at least three days of the week for at least three months (20,23)
Obesity[a]	Body mass index ≥30 kg · m^{-2} or waist girth >102 cm (40 inches) for men and >88 cm (35 inches) for women (2)
Hypertension	Systolic blood pressure ≥140 mmHg and/or diastolic ≥90 mmHg, confirmed by measurements on at least two separate occasions, or on antihypertensive medication (10)
Dyslipidemia	Low-density lipoprotein (LDL-C) cholesterol ≥130 mg · dL^{-1} (3.37 mmol · L^{-1}) or high-density lipoprotein (HDL-C) cholesterol ≤40 mg · dL^{-1} (1.04 mmol· L^{-1}) or on lipid-lowering medication. If total serum cholesterol is all that is available use ≥200 mg · dL^{-1} (5.18 mmol · L^{-1}) (3)
Prediabetes	Impaired fasting glucose (IFG) = fasting plasma glucose ≥100 mg · dL^{-1} (5.50 mmol · L^{-1}) but <126 mg · dL^{-1} (6.93 mmol · L^{-1}) or impaired glucose tolerance (IGT) = 2-hour values in oral glucose tolerance test (OGTT) ≥140 mg · dL^{-1} (7.70 mmol · L^{-1}) but <200 mg · dL^{-1} (11.00 mmol · L^{-1}) confirmed by measurements on at least two separate occasions (1)

NEGATIVE RISK FACTOR	DEFINING CRITERIA
High-serum HDL cholesterol[†]	≥60 mg · dL^{-1} (1.55 mmol · L^{-1})

Note: It is common to sum risk factors in making clinical judgments. If HDL is high, subtract one risk factor from the sum of positive risk factors, because high HDL decreases CVD risk.

[a]Professional opinions vary regarding the most appropriate markers and thresholds for obesity; therefore, allied health professionals should use clinical judgment when evaluating this risk factor.

Adapted from American College of Sports Medicine. *ACSM's Guidelines for Exercise Testing and Prescription,* 8th ed. Philadelphia (PA): Wolters Kluwer Health Ltd: 2009, 28 p.

has experienced chest pain. The key features that classify this pain as *favoring an is-chemic origin* are the *character* of the pain, the *location* of the pain, and the factors associated with *provoking* the pain. It is important to ask the client to describe the feeling with as little prompting for specific characteristics as possible. Ideally, you want the client to describe the feeling using self-selected words. Asking a client to describe the location of the pain is better than asking if there is pain in the shoulders, neck, or arms.

Recommendations for a Medical Examination

In 1998, the American Heart Association (AHA) and the ACSM published a preparticipation screening questionnaire, found in Figure 2.4, for use in health and fitness program facilities (2). This questionnaire, which mirrors the ACSM risk stratification process, is presented in a simplified, checklist-type response format. The top section, which asks about disease history and signs and symptoms, would identify a person at

TABLE 2.3. MAJOR SIGNS OR SYMPTOMS SUGGESTIVE OF CARDIOVASCULAR, PULMONARY, OR METABOLIC DISEASE[a]

SIGN OR SYMPTOM	CLARIFICATION/SIGNIFICANCE
Pain, discomfort (or other anginal equivalent) in the chest, neck, jaw, arms, or other areas that may result from ischemia	One of the cardinal manifestations of cardiac disease, particular coronary artery disease Key features *favoring an ischemic origin* include: • *Character:* Constricting, squeezing, burning, "heaviness" or "heavy feeling" • *Location:* Substernal, across midthorax, anteriorly; in one or both arms, shoulders; in neck, cheeks, teeth; in forearms, fingers in interscapular region • *Provoking factors:* Exercise or exertion, excitement, other forms of stress, cold weather, occurrence after meals Key features *against an ischemic origin* include: • *Character:* Dull ache; "knifelike," sharp, stabbing; "jabs" aggravated by respiration • *Location:* In left submammary area; in left hemithorax • *Provoking factors:* After completion of exercise, provoked by a specific body motion
Shortness of breath at rest or with mild exertion	Dyspnea (defined as an abnormally uncomfortable awareness of breathing) is one of the principal symptoms of cardiac and pulmonary disease. It commonly occurs during strenuous exertion in healthy, well-trained persons and during moderate exertion in healthy, untrained persons. However, it should be regarded as abnormal when it occurs at a level of exertion that is not expected to evoke this symptom in a given individual. Abnormal exertional dyspnea suggests the presence of cardiopulmonary disorders, in particular left ventricular dysfunction or chronic obstructive pulmonary disease.
Dizziness or syncope	Syncope (defined as a loss of consciousness) is most commonly caused by a reduced perfusion of the brain. Dizziness and, in particular, syncope *during* exercise may result from cardiac disorders that prevent the normal rise (or an actual fall) in cardiac output. Such cardiac disorders are potentially life-threatening and include severe coronary artery disease, hypertrophic cardiomyopathy, aortic stenosis, and malignant ventricular dysrhythmias. Although dizziness or syncope shortly *after* cessation of exercise should not be ignored, these symptoms may occur even in healthy persons as a result of a reduction in venous return to the heart.
Orthopnea or paroxysmal nocturnal dyspnea	Orthopnea refers to dyspnea occurring at rest in the recumbent position that is relieved promptly by sitting upright or standing. Paroxysmal nocturnal dyspnea refers to dyspnea, beginning usually 2–5 h after the onset of sleep, which may be relieved by sitting on the side of the bed or getting out of bed. Both are symptoms of left ventricular dysfunction. Although nocturnal dyspnea may occur in persons with chronic obstructive pulmonary disease, it differs in that it is usually relieved after the person relieves himself or herself of secretions rather than specifically by sitting up.
Ankle edema	Bilateral ankle edema that is most evident at night is a characteristic sign of heart failure or bilateral chronic venous insufficiency. Unilateral edema of a limb often results from venous thrombosis or lymphatic blockage in the limb. Generalized edema (known as anasarca) occurs in persons with the nephrotic syndrome, severe heart failure, or hepatic cirrhosis.

(continued)

TABLE 2.3. MAJOR SIGNS OR SYMPTOMS SUGGESTIVE OF CARDIOVASCULAR, PULMONARY, OR METABOLIC DISEASE[a] (Continued)

SIGN OR SYMPTOM	CLARIFICATION/SIGNIFICANCE
Palpitations or tachycardia	Palpitations (defined as an unpleasant awareness of the forceful or rapid beating of the heart) may be induced by various disorders of cardiac rhythm. These include tachycardia, bradycardia of sudden onset, ectopic beats, compensatory pauses, and accentuated stroke volume resulting from valvular regurgitation. Palpitations also often result from anxiety states and high cardiac output (or hyperkinetic) states, such as anemia, fever, thyrotoxicosis, arteriovenous fistula, and the so-called idiopathic hyperkinetic heart syndrome.
Intermittent claudication	Intermittent claudication refers to the pain that occurs in a muscle with an inadequate blood supply (usually as a result of atherosclerosis) that is stressed by exercise. The pain does not occur with standing or sitting, is reproducible from day to day, is more severe when walking upstairs or up a hill, and is often described as a cramp, which disappears within 1–2 min after stopping exercise. Coronary artery disease is more prevalent in persons with intermittent claudication. Patients with diabetes are at increased risk for this condition.
Known heart murmur	Although some may be innocent, heart murmurs may indicate valvular or other cardiovascular disease. From an exercise safety standpoint, it is especially important to exclude hypertrophic cardiomyopathy and aortic stenosis as underlying causes because these are among the more common causes of exertion-related sudden cardiac death.
Unusual fatigue or shortness of breath with usual activities	Although there may be benign origins for these symptoms, they also may signal the onset of, or change in the status of cardiovascular, pulmonary, or metabolic disease.

[a]These signs or symptoms must be interpreted within the clinical context in which they appear because they are not all specific for cardiovascular, pulmonary, or metabolic disease.

Adapted from American College of Sports Medicine. *ACSM's Guidelines for Exercise Testing and Prescription*, 8th ed. Philadelphia (PA): Wolters Kluwer Health Ltd: 2009, 26–27 p.

high risk. The appropriate recommendation would be that persons considered high risk should not participate in an HRPF assessment involving exercise until cleared for participation by a physician. The client's physician may refer the individual to a medically supervised facility for the assessment if exercise is deemed appropriate. The middle section, which asks about risk factors, seeks to identify those with multiple risk factors (moderate-risk stratification) and recommends consulting with a physician or other appropriate healthcare provider prior to performing any HRPF assessments that involve exercise. The physician may refer such an individual to a facility with a professionally qualified staff for the assessment if exercise is deemed appropriate. The bottom section of the form, which allows the client to designate that none of the above applies (low-risk stratification), suggests that the individual is an appropriate candidate for the HRPF assessment without any consultation with a healthcare provider. The *GETP8* provides a flow chart to aid in decision making about the need for a medical examination, which was shown in Figure 2.2. Keep in mind: The level of intensity of any exercise to be performed should guide decisions related to HRPF assessments.

Contraindications for Exercise

It is also critically important to recognize that a client may have medical conditions for which exercise should not be performed until the condition is resolved. These are

AHA/ACSM Health/Fitness Facility Preparticipation Screening Questionnaire

Assess your health status by marking all *true* statements

History

You have had

_____ a heart attack

_____ heart surgery

_____ cardiac catheterization

_____ coronary angioplasty (PTCA)

_____ pacemaker/implantable cardiac
       defibrillator/rhythm disturbance

_____ heart valve disease

_____ heart failure

_____ heart transplantation

_____ congenital heart disease

*If you marked any of these statements in this section, consult your physician or other appropriate healthcare provider before engaging in exercise. You may need to use a facility with a **medically qualified staff.***

Symptoms

_____ You experience chest discomfort with exertion.

_____ You experience unreasonable breathlessness.

_____ You experience dizziness, fainting, or blackouts.

_____ You take heart medications.

Other health issues

_____ You have diabetes.

_____ You have asthma or other lung disease.

_____ You have burning or cramping sensations in your lower
       legs when walking short distances.

_____ You have musculoskeletal problems that limit your
       physical activity.

_____ You have concerns about the safety of exercise.

_____ You take prescription medication(s).

_____ You are pregnant.

Cardiovascular risk factors

_____ You are a man older than 45 years.

_____ You are a women older than 55 years, have had a
       hysterectomy, or are postmenopausal.

_____ You smoke, or quit smoking within the previous 6 months.

_____ Your blood pressure is >140/90 mm Hg.

_____ You do not know your blood pressure.

_____ You take blood pressure medication.

_____ Your blood cholesterol level is >200 mg/dL.

_____ You do not know your cholesterol level.

_____ You have a close blood relative who had a heart attack or
       heart surgery before age 55 (father or brother) or age 65
       (mother or sister).

_____ You are physically inactive (i.e., you get <30 minutes of
       moderate-intensity physical activity on at least 3 days per week).

_____ You are >20 pounds overweight.

*If you marked two or more of the statements in this section you should consult your physician or other appropriate healthcare provider before engaging in exercise. You might benefit from using a facility with a **professionally qualified exercise staff**[†] to guide your exercise program.*

_____ None of the above

You should be able to exercise safely without consulting your physician or other appropriate healthcare provider in a self-guided program or almost any facility that meets your exercise program needs.

*Modified from American College of Sports Medicine and American Heart Association. ACSM/AHA joint position statement: recommendations for cardiovascular screening, staffing, and emergency policies at health/fitness facilities. *Med Sci Sports Exerc.* 1998;30:1009–18.

[†]Professionally qualified exercise staff refers to appropriately trained individuals who possess academic training, practical and clinical knowlege, skills, and abilities commensurate with the credentials defined in Appendix D, *Guidelines for Exercise Training and Prescription* (8th ed.).

FIGURE 2.4. American Heart Association (AHA)/American College of Sports Medicine (ACSM) Health/Fitness Facility Preparticipation Screening Questionnaire. (Adapted from American College of Sports Medicine. *ACSM's Guidelines for Exercise Testing and Prescription,* 8th ed. Philadelphia [PA] : Wolters Kluwer Health Ltd: 2009, 21 p.)

conditions for which the immediate risks of exercise outweigh any potential benefit that could be derived from the exercise. These are called contraindications for exercise and are listed in Box 2.2. Clients identified with these factors should not perform an HRPF assessment and should be informed to seek medical attention for the condition.

OTHER HEALTH ISSUES TO CONSIDER

It is important to recognize that the ACSM and AHA screening recommendations are focused mostly on cardiovascular risk issues. If the screening identifies a medical history of musculoskeletal problems, then a similar referral to a healthcare provider should be made before any HRPF assessments that could impact the musculoskeletal condition.

UNDERSTANDING MEDICATION USAGE

A list of all medications that a client is presently using should be obtained during the preassessment screening. It is beyond the level of expertise for a nonclinical exercise professional to have a complete understanding of all medications. However, the fitness professional should minimally know if a client is taking any medications and whether the medication may alter the client's response to acute or chronic exercise. There are many sources to review medications, their side effects, and how they impact the exercise response. Some of these may get quite involved and are beyond the scope of information needed by the fitness professional. One good Internet source is provided by the National Institutes of Health (NIH; http://www.nlm.nih.gov/medlineplus/druginformation.html).

The *GETP8* provides two appendices (A1 and A2) on medications. The first provides a list of medication names by drug classification and the second provides effects of each medication class on exercise blood pressure, heart rate, and exercise capacity. This information is important, particularly for assessments of cardiorespiratory fitness that require measurements of heart rate during the exercise test.

The fitness professional should not instruct a client to stop taking or change the timing of his or her medication prior to any HRPF assessment. Only the client's physician should make such decisions.

SUMMARY

Preassessment screening includes informed consent, risk stratification, and determination of the recommendations for a medical evaluation prior to performing the HRPF assessment. The informed consent is a process that involves several key elements to allow the client to completely understand the essential factors related to performing the HRPF assessment. The risk stratification helps the fitness professional guide the client in making decisions about health readiness to proceed with the HRPF assessment. Depending on the client's risk level, a referral to the client's health care provider may be important prior to proceeding with the assessment.

RISK STRATIFICATION USING A COMPREHENSIVE HEALTH HISTORY QUESTIONNAIRE

Data Collection
Ask a friend or relative over the age of 45 to complete the comprehensive HHQ (be sure to omit a name or any identifying information with your assignment). Review the questionnaire with this individual.

Written Report
Determine this person's ACSM risk stratification classification. Provide the criteria for the selection of the correct ACSM risk stratification classification.

RISK STRATIFICATION USING THE AHA/ACSM HEALTH/ FITNESS FACILITY PREPARTICIPATION SCREENING QUESTIONNAIRE

Data Collection
Ask a friend or relative over the age of 45 to complete the AHA/ACSM Health/Fitness Facility Preparticipation Screening Questionnaire (be sure to omit a name or any identifying information with your assignment).

Written Report
Based on the results, explain whether this person would be a candidate for completing an HRPF assessment of cardiorespiratory fitness.

ADMINISTERING AN INFORMED CONSENT

In-class Project
With a laboratory partner, practice verbally reviewing the key elements of an informed consent and providing an explanation of procedures for a body composition assessment.

> > > **CASE STUDY**

Todd is a 44-year-old electrical engineer who works 50–60 hours per week. He is 5'9", 233 pounds, with total cholesterol of 192 mg · dL^{-1}, low-density lipo-protein (LDL) of 138 mg · dL^{-1}, high-density lipoprotein (HDL) of 41 mg · dL^{-1}, triglycerides of 200 mg · dL^{-1}, and blood glucose of 120 mg · dL^{-1}. Todd's rest-ing heart rate is 81 bpm and blood pressure is 144/86 mmHg. His waist and hip circumference measures are 42 inches and 40 inches, respectively. Todd has never smoked, but usually has one to two glasses of wine with dinner. He reports no leisure-time physical activity and does not exercise on a regular basis (less than two sessions per month). Todd denies all complaints of chest discom-fort and shortness of breath at rest or with exertion; however, he has gained 20 pounds over the last 2 years. Todd's wife reports he snores frequently and has difficulty waking up in the mornings. Further testing reveals that Todd has obstructive sleep apnea and is being treated with continuous positive airway pressure (CPAP). A review of his family history reveals that Todd's father had double-bypass surgery at age 53 and suffered a fatal myocardial infarction at age 62. Todd's brother (42 years old) also is hypertensive and was recently diag-nosed with type 2 diabetes, which is being treated with diet and physical activity recommendations. Todd has been referred to your facility for coronary artery disease risk factor reduction and physical activity counseling.

Determine the presence or absence of each CVD risk factor, any signs or symptoms, the ACSM risk stratification, the recommendations for a medical exam and exercise test, and the recommendation for physician supervision of the exercise test.

REFERENCES

1. American Diabetes Association. Diagnosis and Classification of Diabetes Mellitus. *Diabetes Care.* 2007; 30(suppl 1):S42–7.
2. Balady GJ, Chaitman B, Driscoll D, et al. American College of Sports Medicine and American Heart Asso-ciation joint position statement: recommendations for cardiovascular screening, staffing, and emergency procedures at health/fitness facilities. *Med Sci Sports Exerc.* 1998;30:1009–18.
3. U.S. Department of Health and Human Services and Centers for Disease Control and Prevention. *Physical Activity and Health: A Report of the Surgeon General.* Atlanta (GA) 1996: National Center for Chronic Dis-ease Prevention and Health Promotion.

Risk Factor Assessments

RESTING BLOOD PRESSURE

Blood pressure (BP) is the force of blood against the walls of the arteries and veins created by the heart as it pumps blood to every part of the body. For a health risk assessment, arterial BP is measured and expressed in units of millimeters of mercury (mmHg). Two phases of BP, systolic and diastolic, are assessed. The systolic BP is the maximum pressure in the arteries during the contraction (systole) phase of the heart. Diastolic BP is the minimum pressure in the arteries during the relaxation (diastole) phase of the heart. BP measurements are used in risk stratification, as was discussed in Chapter 2, and contribute to the decision-making process regarding the appropriateness of performing a vigorous to maximal exercise test (see Fig. 2.2).

MEASUREMENT

The direct measure of BP requires placement of a catheter in an artery followed by the insertion of a pressure transducer into the catheter. Obviously, this is an invasive procedure that can only be performed by trained clinical professionals. Although often used during surgical operations and within research settings, the direct method is not required for determining resting BP in routine healthcare practice. Resting BP is typically assessed by employing an indirect method termed auscultation. Auscultation involves listening to internal sounds of the body using a stethoscope. For BP assessment, a stethoscope is placed over an artery to listen for the sounds of Korotkoff on the arterial walls. The five phases of the Korotkoff sounds are provided in Box 3.1. The sounds of Korotkoff heard through the stethoscope during the BP measurement come from the turbulence of blood in the artery, which is caused by blood moving from an area of higher pressure to an area of lower pressure. A cuff is applied to the upper arm and is inflated with air pressure by pumping up a hand bulb. This air pressure inside the BP cuff occludes the blood flow within the brachial artery. As long as the pressure in the cuff is higher than the systolic BP, the artery remains occluded or collapsed and no sound is heard through the applied stethoscope. When the air pressure is slowly released from

BOX 3.1	Korotkoff Sounds

- Phase 1. The first, initial sound or the onset of sound. Sounds like clear, repetitive tapping. The sound may be faint at first and gradually increase in intensity or volume to phase 2.
- Phase 2. Sounds like a soft tapping or murmur. The sounds are often longer than the phase 1 sounds. These sounds have also been described as having a swishing component. The phase 2 sounds are typically 10–15 mmHg after the onset of sound (phase 1).
- Phase 3. Sounds like a loud tapping sound; high in both pitch and intensity. These sounds are crisper and louder than the phase 2 sounds.
- Phase 4. Sounds like a muffling of the sound. The sounds become less distinct and less audible. Another way of describing this sound is as soft or blowing.
- Phase 5. Sounds like the complete disappearance of sound. The true disappearance of sound usually occurs within 8–10 mmHg of the muffling of sound (phase 4).

the cuff, the pressure inside the cuff will eventually equal the driving pressure of the blood in the artery and the first sound will be heard in the stethoscope. This sound corresponds to the measure of systolic BP. As the pressure in the cuff continues to drop, it will eventually get to a point where the cuff is no longer occluding the artery and all sounds will disappear. The pressure reading at the last sound heard is the diastolic BP.

Measurement Equipment

BP measurement using the ausculatory method requires a stethoscope, a manometer or sphygmomanometer (a device to measure pressure), and a cuff with an inflatable bladder that is wrapped around the limb (typically the arm). The two common types of manometers used for BP measurement are mercury and aneroid as shown in Figure 3.1. Mercury, the standard for pressure measurements, is housed in a small reservoir (~300 mm) located at the base of a vertical glass column. However, because mercury is a toxic chemical, aneroid sphygmomanometers are becoming more common in the workplace. Indeed, many facilities have instituted a ban on all devices containing mercury. Aneroid sphygmomanometers measure the pressure by the movement of a spring-loaded needle that moves on a dial-type scale. Facilities should have at least three different BP cuff sizes available: small, medium, and large. There are index lines on many of the newer sphygmomanometer cuffs to help determine the correct cuff for a client's arm circumference. Typically, the appropriate BP bladder should encircle at least 80% of the arm's circumference without overlapping. In general, a cuff that is too small will

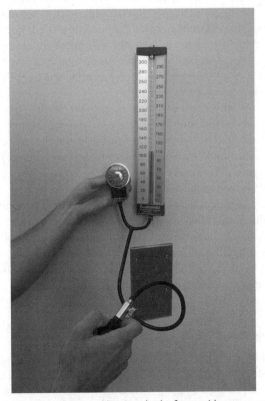

FIGURE 3.1. A Y-tube is used to perform a calibration check of anaeroid manometers.

result in an overestimation of BP and a cuff that is too long will result in an underestimation of BP.

Equipment used in the measurement of BP is widely available commercially but varies greatly in quality. Sphygmomanometer units can be purchased in most drug stores, various health and fitness commercial catalogs, and medical supply stores. A high-quality stethoscope is worth the investment to help in hearing clear Korotkoff sounds.

Automated Systems

Electronic BP machines have been available for many years, and industrial models are increasingly being used in both hospitals and doctors' offices. Commercial models have also become relatively inexpensive for individuals to perform self-monitoring of BP at home (11). Most of these systems use the oscillatory method for measuring BP. This method uses a cuff that fills with a fluid, instead of air. Systolic BP is detected when oscillations begin during the deflation of the pressure, with diastolic BP being recorded at the point of maximal oscillations. Although these devices have been shown to provide reasonably accurate BP measurements, they are limited by a lack of a simple and inexpensive method to verify their calibration over time.

Calibration of an Aneroid Manometer

The aneroid manometer needs to be checked regularly for accuracy against the standard mercury manometer. Because this calibration check procedure requires only a few minutes, it is reasonable to suggest that this procedure be performed daily, and it should always be done if the aneroid manometer was dropped or jostled. For this reason alone, it is recommended that facilities keep at least one mercury manometer. The set-up of the calibration system is shown in Figure 3.1 and simply consists of a Y tube with the bottom end attached to a hand bulb and the top ends attached to both manometers. Note that the standard here is the mercury manometer.

The first step is to verify that both manometers are reading zero when there is no pressure being applied to the hand bulb. The next step in the process involves gently pumping the hand bulb so that the pressure reads 200 mmHg on the mercury manometer. At this point, the reading of the aneroid manometer is recorded. The pressure is then released in approximately 30-mmHg increments (i.e., 170, 140, 110, 80, 50) with simultaneous recordings being made at each interval.

If the readings are identical between the two manometers, the aneroid unit is considered perfectly calibrated. If there is a difference between the two manometers and the difference is consistent, the aneroid unit can still be used with a correction factor (e.g., if there was always a reading of 6 mmHg more for the aneroid gauge, then readings made with this unit would need to have 6 mmHg subtracted). If, however, the readings between the two manometers are variable and >4 mmHg, then the aneroid unit should not be used until it is repaired.

Assessment Technique

For accurate resting BP readings, it is important that the client be made as comfortable as possible. There exists what is called the white coat syndrome in the measurement of BP, as with many other physiologic and psychological measures taken on people. This white coat syndrome refers to an elevation of BP because of the effect of being in a doctor's

BOX 3.2	Procedures for Assessment of Resting Blood Pressure

1. Patients should be seated quietly for at least 5 minutes in a chair with back support (rather than on an examination table) with their feet on the floor and their arm supported at heart level. Patients should refrain from smoking cigarettes or ingesting caffeine during the 30 minutes preceding the measurement.
2. Measuring supine and standing values may be indicated under special circumstances.
3. Wrap cuff firmly around upper arm at heart level; align cuff with brachial artery.
4. The appropriate cuff size must be used to ensure accurate measurement. The bladder within the cuff should encircle at least 80% of the upper arm. Many adults require a large adult cuff.
5. Place stethoscope bell below the antecubital space over the brachial artery.
6. Quickly inflate cuff pressure to 20 mmHg above first Korotkoff sound.
7. Slowly release pressure at rate equal to 2 to 5 mmHg per second.
8. Systolic BP is the point at which the first of two or more Korotkoff sounds is heard (phase 1) and diastolic BP is the point before the disappearance of Korotkoff sounds (phase 5).
9. At least two measurements should be made (minimum of 1 minute apart).
10. Provide to patients, verbally and in writing, their specific BP numbers and BP goals.

American College of Sports Medicine. *ACSM's Guidelines for Exercise Testing and Prescription*, 8th ed. Philadelphia (PA): Wolters Kluwer Health Ltd: 2009, 46 p.

Modified from National High Blood Pressure Education Program. *The Seventh Report of the Joint National Committee on Prevention, Detection, Evaluation, and Treatment of High Blood Pressure (JNC7)*. Washington, DC: 2003; 03-5233. For additional, more detailed recommendations, see Pickering TG, Hall JE, Appel LJ, et al. Recommendations for blood pressure measurement in humans and experimental animals. *Hypertension*. 2005;45:142–61.

office or in a clinical setting (i.e., clinician wearing a white lab coat). The recommended procedures for assessing resting BP are listed in Box 3.2. The American Heart Association has recommended measuring both right and left arm BPs at the initial evaluation and then choosing the arm with the higher pressure for all subsequent assessments.

When an individual is beginning to learn the skill of BP measurement, it is helpful to work with an experienced technician who can listen with the trainee by using a dual head (two sets of listening tubes/earpieces) or teaching stethoscope as shown in Figure 3.2. Some helpful technique tips are as follows:

- Ideally, the client cuff should be applied to bare skin. However, if clothing on the arm is thin where the stethoscope is placed, it should not interfere with the measurement except for the slightly lower intensity of the sound. If the clothing is worn and it is difficult to hear the Korotkoff sounds, then the procedure should be repeated with the arm bared.
- Locate the client's brachial artery (position with the palm up and arm rotated outward on the thumb side with the arm hyperextended). This artery, and thus pulse, is just medial to the biceps tendon. Mark the artery with an appropriate marker (water color) for the stethoscope bell placement, especially if the BP will be assessed again during exercise.

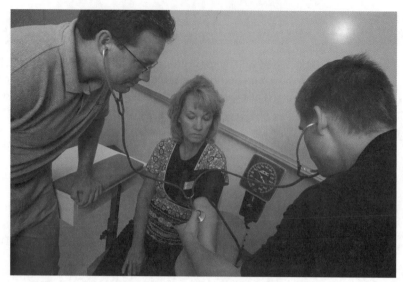

FIGURE 3.2. Use of a double-headed stethoscope used for training technicians learning to measure blood pressure.

- Firmly place the bell of the stethoscope over the artery. Do not place the bell of the stethoscope under the lip of the BP cuff.
- The stethoscope earpieces should be facing forward, toward the nose, in the same direction as the ear canal. (Note: If a stethoscope is being shared, the earpieces should be cleaned between users.)
- Position the manometer (either mercury or aneroid) so that the manometer is clearly visible and at eye level to avoid any parallax (distortion from looking up or down) error.
- After identifying the systolic BP, the pressure can be lowered ≈20 mmHg rapidly and then slowed to the standard deflation rate of 2–5 mmHg per second. More rapid deflation leads to errors in the identification of diastolic BP.
- Record both the fourth and fifth phase sounds if clearly heard. Always record only even numbers and round off upward to the nearest 2 mmHg. Always continue to listen for any BP sounds for at least 10 mmHg below the fifth phase.
- Increase the intensity, or loudness, of the sounds of Korotkoff by having the client raise the arm and rapidly make a fist and relax 5–10 times.

INTERPRETATION

As noted in Table 2.2, the criteria for the hypertension risk factor are a systolic BP of ≥140 mmHg and/or a diastolic BP of ≥90 mmHg. Remember that high readings need to be confirmed by at least one other reading on a separate day. Also note that only physicians can make a diagnosis of hypertension. Fitness professionals should inform clients if their blood pressure is elevated in the hypertensive range and recommend that they follow up with their healthcare provider.

More detailed classifications of resting BP readings are found in Table 3.1. These classifications, which are from the Seventh Report of the National High Blood Pressure Education Program (3), also contain recommendations for patient follow-up. Fitness professionals should be familiar with at least the recommendations contained in the Executive Summary of this report.

TABLE 3.1. CLASSIFICATION AND MANAGEMENT OF BLOOD PRESSURE FOR ADULTS[a]

BP CLASSI-FICATION	SBP mmHg	DPB mmHg	LIFESTYLE MODIFICA-TION	INITIAL DRUG THERAPY WITHOUT COMPELLING INDICATION	WITH COMPELLING INDICATIONS
Normal	<120	And <80	Encourage		
Prehypertension	120–139	Or 80–89	Yes	No anti-hypertensive drug indicated	Drug(s) for compelling indications[b]
Stage 1 hypertension	140–159	Or 90–99	Yes	Antihypertensive drug(s) indicated	Drug(s) for compelling indications[b]
					Other antihypertensive drugs, as needed
Stage 2 hypertension	≥160	Or ≥100	Yes	Antihypertensive drug(s) indicated Two-drug combination for most[c]	

(140/90) 3

BP, blood pressure; DBP, diastolic blood pressure; SBP, systolic blood pressure.

[a]Treatment determined by highest BP category.

[b]Compelling indications include heart failure, post–myocardial infarction, high coronary heart disease risk, diabetes, chronic kidney disease, and recurrent stroke prevention. Treat patients with chronic kidney disease or diabetes to BP goal of <130/80 mmHg.

[c]Initial combined therapy should be used cautiously in those at risk for orthostatic hypotension.

American College of Sports Medicine. *ACSM's Guidelines for Exercise Testing and Prescription*, 8th ed. Philadelphia (PA): Wolters Kluwer Health Ltd: 2009, 47 p.

Adapted from National High Blood Pressure Education Program. *The Seventh Report of the Joint National Committee on Prevention, Detection, Evaluation, and Treatment of High Blood Pressure (JNC7)*. JAMA. 2003; 289:2560–72.

BLOOD TESTS

To determine the presence of two of the coronary disease risk factors, hypercholesterolemia and prediabetes, a recent fasted blood test is required. Some clients who obtain regular physical examinations from their physicians may have had a recent test. If so, this value can be used for the risk stratification. If the client does not recall the exact test values, a copy of the blood test report may need to be acquired from the healthcare provider.

Unfortunately, many American adults do not know their cholesterol and glucose values and thus would need to obtain a test. In fact, some surveys performed in 2004 reported that 4 in 10 Americans with heart disease risk factors did not know their cholesterol level and 7 in 10 Americans did not know their blood glucose level (2,8). The fitness professional has a couple of simple solutions if values are unknown. One, a contract with a local laboratory that provides these blood-testing services can be obtained and then clients can be referred to this facility for testing. Another variation is to actually collect the blood sample from the client and then send the sample to the laboratory for analysis. The second option is to actually purchase the instrumentation for performing these tests. Many small, relatively economical systems, which are available commercially, offer the ability to perform cholesterol and glucose testing (and possibly other useful tests). Then both collection and testing of the sample can be performed on-site. Generally, such results are available for interpretation within minutes.

BLOOD SAMPLING METHODS

Phlebotomy is the practice of withdrawing blood from a blood vessel into a blood collection tube. Typically this is done either by inserting a needle into a vein (larger-volume sample) or by puncturing a finger (smaller-volume sample). The venipuncture method is obviously more involved and thus requires a skilled phlebotomist to perform the task. There are professional phlebotomy training courses available as this skill is needed in all medical facilities and can involve advanced skills such as starting intravenous access lines, obtaining samples from arteries, and drawing samples from infants, children, and adults with characteristics that make the blood draw challenging. Fortunately, the sample needed for the cholesterol and glucose measures only requires drawing a sample from an arm vein. There are modified courses that can provide training limited to this purpose. Some states have regulations that restrict the practice of phlebotomy to those with a defined level of training; thus, the state department of health should be contacted to determine if training and licensing regulations exist.

For facilities that purchase their own mini-sample systems, the blood sample can be obtained by a finger puncture as shown in Figure 3.3. This skill is much simpler and requires

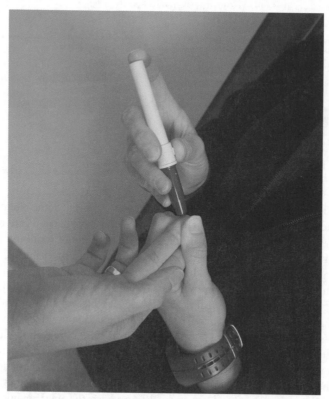

FIGURE 3.3. A device used to puncture the finger to obtain a blood sample. Note: Protective gloves would be worn by the technician.

less training. In most cases an automated device is placed on the finger and then triggered to puncture the skin. Indeed, all individuals with diabetes are trained to perform this technique, as they need to regularly self-monitor their blood glucose levels. The sample may be collected into a small capillary tube or the drop of blood that forms on the finger may be applied directly to a reagent pad depending on the instrumentation used.

STANDARD PRECAUTIONS

All healthcare and allied healthcare professionals should be trained to protect themselves against exposure to bloodborne pathogens. Indeed, the Occupational Safety and Health Administration (OSHA) of the Department of Labor has set national standards for these protections called Standard Precautions. The federal law (29 CFR 1910.1030) was enacted in 1991 and provides the requirements for training and regular reviews of the procedures that should be followed to protect employees from the risks of exposure to bloodborne pathogens (14). Certainly all workers who will be involved in handling blood are required to have this training. However, it is reasonable for all fitness professionals who work with clients to assume they may be at risk of exposure to blood (e.g., an accident that results in a cut of the skin) or possibly other bodily fluids (with the exception of sweat). Thus, it is prudent for all fitness professionals to obtain training in Standard Precautions.

INTERPRETATION

Regardless of how the fitness professional obtains the blood test information, it is important to know how to interpret the results. The National Cholesterol Education Program has standardized the interpretation of results of cholesterol, including high-density lipoprotein (HDL), low-density lipoprotein (LDL), and triglycerides (7). Table 3.2 provides these classifications. Refer back to Chapter 2 for the criteria for the positive risk factor of hypercholesterolemia and the negative risk factor of high HDL. Likewise, the American Diabetes Association has set the standards that have become uniformly accepted in healthcare for interpretation of fasting blood glucose (1). The risk factor criteria (prediabetes) are values from $100-125$ mg $\cdot$ dL^{-1}. Values <100 mg $\cdot$ dL^{-1} are considered normal and values ≥ 126 mg $\cdot$ dL^{-1} are considered diagnostic for diabetes. Remember, as with resting blood pressure measures, elevated values should be confirmed by at least one other test.

OBESITY

Obesity was once thought to only affect coronary artery disease (CAD) through its impact on the other risk factors such as diabetes, hypertension, and hyperlipidemia. In other words, obesity was considered to be a primary factor leading to diabetes, hypertension, and hyperlipidemia, but only a secondary factor for CAD. This changed in 1998 when the American Heart Association, based on its review of the scientific literature, declared that obesity should be considered a major, independent risk factor for CAD (4).

Obesity is defined as an excessive amount of body fat. The assessment of body composition, which involves estimating body fat percentage, is the focus of Chapter 4 of this manual. From a risk factor assessment perspective, obesity is determined from evaluating an individual's body weight compared to his or her height and also considering the girth of the abdominal region of the body. The term *overweight* is used as classification

TABLE 3.2. ATP III CLASSIFICATION OF LDL, TOTAL, AND HDL CHOLESTEROL (mg · dL^{-1})

LDL CHOLESTEROL

<100[a]	Optimal
100–129	Near optimal/above optimal
130–159	Borderline high
160–189	High
≥190	Very high

TOTAL CHOLESTEROL

<200	Desirable
200–239	Borderline high
≥240	High

HDL CHOLESTEROL

<40	Low
≥60	High

TRIGLYCERIDES

<150	Normal
150–199	Borderline high
200–499	High
≥500	Very high

LDL, low-density lipoprotein; HDL, high-density lipoprotein.

[a]According to the American Heart Association/American College of Cardiology 2006 update (endorsed by the National Heart, Lung, and Blood Institute), it is reasonable to treat LDL cholesterol to <70 mg · dL^{-1} (<1.81 mmol · L^{-1}) in patients with coronary and other atherosclerotic vascular disease (12).

NOTE: To convert LDL cholesterol, total cholesterol, and HDL cholesterol from mg · dL^{-1} to mmol · L^{-1}, multiply by 0.0259. To convert triglycerides from mg · dL^{-1} to mmol · L^{-1}, multiply by 0.0113.

American College of Sports Medicine. *ACSM's Guidelines for Exercise Testing and Prescription*, 8th ed. Philadelphia (PA): Wolters Kluwer Health Ltd: 2009, 48 p.

Adapted from National Cholesterol Education Program. *Third Report of the National Cholesterol Education Program (NCEP) Expert Panel on Detection, Evaluation, and Treatment of High Blood Cholesterol in Adults (Adult Treatment Panel III)*. Washington, DC:2002. NIH Publication No. 02-5215.

for body weights that are above what is considered the normal range for one's height, yet below the criteria for obesity.

MEASUREMENT OF HEIGHT AND WEIGHT

Height is measured with an instrument called a stadiometer. A stadiometer consists of a vertical ruler, which is typically mounted to a wall, with a sliding horizontal platform. When mounted to a wall, calibration becomes a moot point because the measurement scale is fixed in place. Portable units and vertical rods attached to weight scales are also available; however, if these are used, then the stadiometer scale readings should be checked with a vertical ruler placed on the platform prior to each measurement session. Although height is a simple and relatively routine measurement to perform, the following important standardization steps as highlighted in Figure 3.4A and B should be used:

- The client must remove shoes and hat (if worn).
- The client should stand erect with feet flat on the floor with heels touching each other.
- If using a wall-mounted stadiometer, the heels, midbody, and upper body parts should be touching the wall.

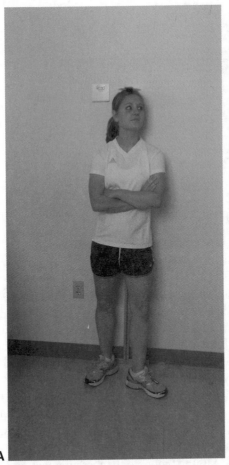 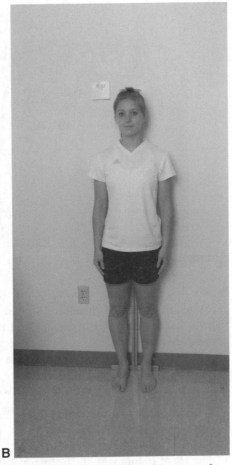

A   B

FIGURE 3.4. **(A)** Incorrect technique used to measure height with a stadiometer; notice shoes are on, feet are not together, head is turned to the side, and the chin is tilted up. **(B)** Correct technique. This is the standardized technique used to measure height with a stadiometer.

- The client should take a normal breath in and hold it while looking straight ahead (head in a neutral position relative to the chin).
- The horizontal headboard should be lowered to touch the top of the head (skull).

Weight can be measured with a variety of types of scales with different mechanisms. One of the most popular types is the balance beam scale. Regardless of the type of scale used, checking the accuracy of the mechanism regularly is important. Most scales provide a method to calibrate the zero point. Checking the scale with no weight on it is an essential step prior to each measurement. If the scale is not reading 0 as shown in Figure 3.5, it should be adjusted to set the reading to 0. Some electronic scales also allow for a measurement of a standard amount of weight as a secondary check for accuracy. Ideally, this standard weight should be in the range of weights you expect for your clients; however, more commonly a smaller amount of weight is used because it is more practical. Some electronic scales may have the ability to adjust the scale if the standardized weight reading is deviant from the scale reading, thereby calibrating the scale at this weight. However, most scales do not have this second adjustment setting and will require professional

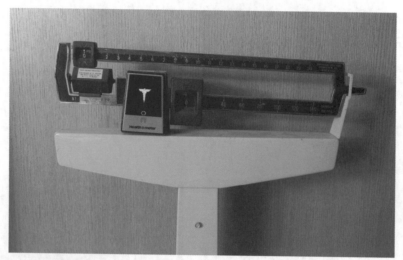

FIGURE 3.5. A balance-beam scale needing calibration of the zero point.

service to make the scale accurate. A calibration check log sheet, recording the date and zero and standard weight readings, should be kept by the fitness professional. The good news is that most high-quality weight scales maintain their calibration quite well. The fitness professional still needs to regularly perform calibration checks to confirm the accuracy of clients' body weight readings. Like height, measuring weight is simple and relatively routine. To obtain accurate measurements, the following important standardization steps as highlighted in Figure 3.6A and B should be used:

- Clients should wear minimal clothing. In fitness assessment programs this is generally considered shorts and a t-shirt (no shoes). However, in other settings with "street clothes" the client should be instructed to remove any multiple layers and empty all pockets.
- The client should void the bladder prior (within 1 hour) to the measurement.
- Ideally, weight should be measured in the morning prior to any meal or beverage consumption. However, because this is not always practical, the time of day should be similar for sequential measurement comparisons with no excess meal and beverage consumption prior to the measurement.

To track body weight over time, it is important to follow the above standardizations. However, for screening programs, variations in the above standards are acceptable with the understanding that the measured weight will be different from the standardized body weight.

Body mass index (BMI), also called the Quetelet Index, is the weight-to-height ratio used to assess the obesity risk factor. This index compares an individual's weight (in kilograms) to his or her height (in meters squared). For example, an individual who weighs 150 pounds and is 68 inches tall would have a BMI calculated as follows:

Convert pounds to kilograms:	150 pounds / 2.2046 pounds/kg = 68.0 kg
Convert inches to centimeters:	68 inches × 2.54 cm/inch = 172.7 cm
Convert centimeters to meters:	172.7 cm / 100 cm/m = 1.727 m
Square the meter measure:	1.727 m × 1.727 m = 2.98 m^2
Calculate BMI:	68.0 kg / 2.98 m^2 = 22.8 kg · m^{-2}

Setting this formula up in a spreadsheet is a simple task and allows fitness professionals the ability to rapidly calculate BMI from height and weight measurements. Also,

Handwritten margin notes:
$BMI = \frac{kg}{m^2}$
$lbs / 2.2 = kg$
$in \times .0254 = m$
$m^2 = m^2$

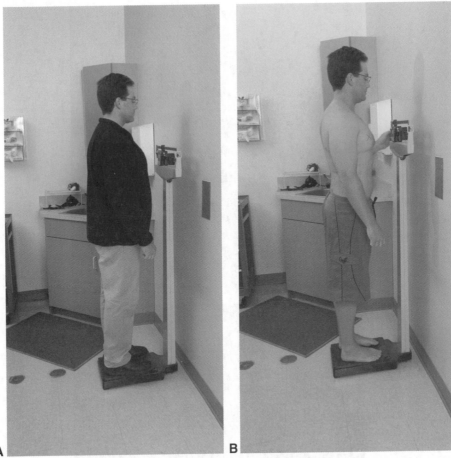

A   B

FIGURE 3.6. (A) Incorrect technique used to measure weight; notice the shoes are on, the patient is fully clothed and wearing a coat. **(B)** Correct standardized technique used to measure weight.

there are many websites such as the one hosted by the Obesity Education Initiative of the National Heart, Lung, and Blood Institute that provide online calculators of BMI (http://www.nhlbisupport.com/bmi/).

MEASUREMENT OF WAIST CIRCUMFERENCE

The pattern of body weight distribution is recognized as an important predictor of health risks of obesity. Thus, the measurement of waist circumference is used as another indicator of obesity. This measurement is used to identify those with the abdominal type of obesity associated with greater health risk. The waist circumference is typically measured at the smallest circumference above the umbilicus and below the xiphoid process. This measurement should be performed using the following important standardization steps as highlighted in Figure 3.7A and B:

- The technician should stand on the right side of the client.
- The measurement should be made on bare skin.
- The measurement should be taken at the end of a normal exhalation by the client.

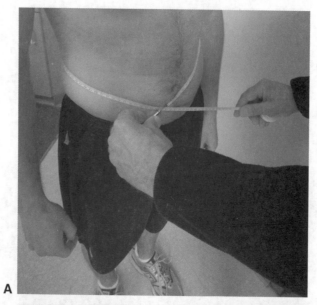

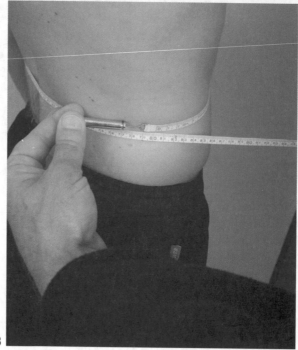

FIGURE 3.7. (A) Incorrect technique used to measure waist circumference; notice the professional is standing in front of the client and the tape is not parallel to the floor. **(B)** Correct standardized technique used to measure waist circumference.

- The measuring tape should be parallel to the floor and should be pulled to lay flat on the skin without compressing the skin (some measurement tapes have a gauge to standardize the tension).
- Multiple measurements should be taken to determine the smallest circumference site. The mean of two measurements at this location (that do not differ by more than 1 cm) is used.

TABLE 3.3. CLASSIFICATION OF DISEASE RISK BASED ON BODY MASS INDEX (BMI) AND WAIST CIRCUMFERENCE

	BMI (kg · m^{-2})	DISEASE RISK[a] RELATIVE TO NORMAL WEIGHT AND WAIST CIRCUMFERENCE	
		MEN, ≤102 cm WOMEN, ≤88 cm	MEN, >102 cm WOMEN, >88 cm
Underweight	<18.5	—	—
Normal	18.5–24.9	—	—
Overweight	25.0–29.9	Increased	High
Obesity, class			
I	30.0–34.9	High	Very high
II	35.0–39.9	Very high	Very high
III	≥40	Extremely high	Extremely high

[a]Disease risk for type 2 diabetes, hypertension, and cardiovascular disease. Dashes (—) indicate that no additional risk at these levels of BMI was assigned. Increased waist circumference can also be a marker for increased risk even in persons of normal weight.

Adapted from American College of Sports Medicine. *ACSM's Guidelines for Exercise Testing and Prescription*, 8th ed. Philadelphia (PA): Wolters Kluwer Health Ltd: 2009, 63 p.

Some have advocated the additional measurement of the hip circumference to assess body fat distribution. The two circumference values are used to determine the waist-to-hip ratio (WHR). The hip circumference is measured as the largest circumference around the buttocks, above the gluteal fold (posterior extension), following the same standardization procedures used for waist measurement.

INTERPRETATION

The classifications for the obesity risk factor were provided in Chapter 2. Note that either (not necessarily both) an elevated BMI (≥30 kg · m^{-2}) or increased waist circumference (>88 cm for women or >102 cm for men) is used as the criterion for the obesity risk factor (9). Additional classifications of BMI status and disease risk can be obtained by using Table 3.3. *ACSM's Guidelines for Exercise Testing and Prescription*, 8th edition (*GETP8*) provides further information on other classifications for the waist circumference and WHR.

It is also important to understand that the BMI scale is not a perfect marker for obesity. Some individuals may have a BMI of <30 kg · m^{-2} and could have excess body fat, and some individuals may have a BMI of ≥30 kg · m^{-2} and could have normal body fat levels. For the latter case, asking a few questions about adult body weight history and involvement in any activities related to heavy lifting (occupational or exercise) should help determine the potential for a misclassification. Clients who report significant weight gain in adulthood without any corresponding increase in heavy lifting activities have probably experienced weight gain composed mostly of body fat and the obesity classification is probably accurate. If significant doubt exists, the client could be referred for a body composition assessment.

PHYSICAL ACTIVITY

Physical activity comprises one of the components of total daily energy expenditure, the other components being resting metabolic rate and the thermic effect of food. The voluntary nature of physical activity makes it the most variable component of total daily energy expenditure. Given the numerous health benefits of regular physical activity

(13), public health guidelines have emerged on the recommended intensity and volume of physical activity necessary to promote health. Specifically, these recommendations advocate a minimum of 30 minutes of moderate-intensity aerobic physical activity on 5 or more days per week or 20 minutes of vigorous-intensity aerobic physical activity on 3 or more days per week (5). They further state that these physical activity targets can be obtained by accumulating bouts of activity throughout the day in smaller increments, such as 8- to 10-minute durations. Given these recommendations, it is important to accurately assess the intensity, frequency, duration, and type of physical activity of an individual. This assessment becomes particularly critical when objectives involve refining the physical activity dose and health response relationship, investigating determinants to physical activity behavior, or evaluating efforts to intervene and increase individual and population levels of physical activity.

From a risk assessment perspective, the highest interest lies in identifying those who are not meeting recommended amounts of physical activity (i.e., inactive or sedentary). Recall from Chapter 2 that the criterion for defining the risk factor of sedentary lifestyle was *not participating in at least 30 minutes of moderate-intensity physical activity on at least 3 days of the week for at least 3 months.* For the most part, the assessment of physical activity can be broken down into either subjective assessment methods or objective assessment methods.

SUBJECTIVE ASSESSMENT

Subjective assessment methods include physical activity questionnaires, diaries, or logs. The level of detail can range from a four-item questionnaire attempting to distinguish overall global levels of activity (low vs. high levels) to a more detailed approach inquiring about different domains of activity (occupational, household, etc.) and the intensity, duration, frequency, and type of activity. There are many questionnaires that have been developed to assess physical activity.

The short version of the International Physical Activity Questionnaire (IPAQ), found in Box 3.3, is one that is relatively simple to use and can be completed by a client in about a minute (6). The instructions are straightforward and the list of examples of physical activities can be modified to fit the background of the client completing the questionnaire. Although the questionnaire offers a choice of "don't know/not sure" for each item, clients should be encouraged to make an estimate of the time for each of the items. The IPAQ uses a variable called metabolic equivalent (MET)·min·week^{-1} for making classifications. MET·min·week^{-1} is calculated by multiplying the MET level for the type of activity by the number of minutes that activity was performed per day by the number of days per week the activity was performed. Walking is scored as 3.3 METs, moderate-intensity activities are scored as 4 METs, and vigorous-intensity activities are scored as 8 METs. For example, a person who reported performing moderate-intensity activity for 30 minutes per day for 5 days of the week would have obtained 600 MET·min·week^{-1} (4 METs × 30 minutes per day × 5 days per week). Physical activity level classifications from the IPAQ assessment are shown in Table 3.4.

OBJECTIVE ASSESSMENT

Objective assessment methods include assessment tools such as motion sensors (i.e., pedometers/step counters and accelerometers as shown in Fig. 3.8), heart rate monitoring, and combination-type approaches (i.e., accelerometer plus heart rate monitoring plus temperature). These types of monitors are typically worn on the body. For instance,

BOX 3.3	International Physical Activity Questionnaire (6)

We are interested in finding out about the kinds of physical activities that people do as part of their everyday lives. The questions will ask you about the time you spent being physically active in the **last 7 days**. Please answer each question even if you do not consider yourself to be an active person. Please think about the activities you do at work, as part of your house and yard work, to get from place to place, and in your spare time for recreation, exercise, or sport.

Think about all the **vigorous** activities that you did in the **last 7 days**. **Vigorous** physical activities refer to activities that take hard physical effort and make you breathe much harder than normal. Think *only* about those physical activities that you did for at least 10 minutes at a time.

1. During the **last 7 days**, on how many days did you do **vigorous** physical activities like heavy lifting, digging, aerobics, or fast bicycling?

   _____ days per week

   ☐ No vigorous physical activities → *Skip to question 3*

2. How much time did you usually spend doing **vigorous** physical activities on one of those days?

   _____ hours per day

   _____ minutes per day

   ☐ Don't know/Not sure

   Think about all the **moderate** activities that you did in the **last 7 days**. **Moderate** activities refer to activities that take moderate physical effort and make you breathe somewhat harder than normal. Think only about those physical activities that you did for at least 10 minutes at a time.

3. During the **last 7 days**, on how many days did you do **moderate** physical activities like carrying light loads, bicycling at a regular pace, or doubles tennis? Do not include walking.

   _____ days per week

   ☐ No moderate physical activities → *Skip to question 5*

4. How much time did you usually spend doing **moderate** physical activities on one of those days?

   _____ hours per day

   _____ minutes per day

   ☐ Don't know/Not sure

   Think about the time you spent **walking** in the **last 7 days**. This includes at work and at home, walking to travel from place to place, and any other walking that you might do solely for recreation, sport, exercise, or leisure.

5. During the **last 7 days**, on how many days did you **walk** for at least 10 minutes at a time?

   _____ days per week

   ☐ No walking → *Skip to question 7*

Box 3.3. continued

6. How much time did you usually spend **walking** on one of those days?

_____ hours per day

_____ minutes per day

☐ Don't know/Not sure

The last question is about the time you spent **sitting** on weekdays during the **last 7 days**. Include time spent at work, at home, while doing course work, and during leisure time. This may include time spent sitting at a desk, visiting friends, reading, or sitting or lying down to watch television.

7. During the **last 7 days**, how much time did you spend **sitting** on a **weekday**?

_____ hours per day

_____ minutes per day

☐ Don't know/Not sure

This is the end of the questionnaire. Thank you for participating.

---

pedometers/step counters and accelerometers can be worn at the level of the hip or ankle, heart rate monitors typically involve wearing a heart rate chest band and a watch-type receiver, and some combination monitors can be worn on the arm or at the hip. Manufacturers of these devices typically specify the chosen location to wear such devices. Objective monitors are usually small, lightweight, and unobtrusive.

The advantages and disadvantages of subjective and objective methods of assessing physical activity are outlined in Table 3.5. In choosing a physical activity assessment tool, be aware of the individual advantages and disadvantages of the method, and match the tool chosen to the needs of the assessment. In most risk stratification situations, it is advantageous to acquire immediate assessment of the client's physical activity behavior. In this instance, a paper questionnaire may be the tool of choice. However, with some advanced planning, objective monitors can be employed. Many facilities now offer assessments with pedometers because of the relatively low cost of these devices and the research evidence that supports their accuracy. To capture the volatile nature of a person's physical activity

---

TABLE 3.4. PHYSICAL ACTIVITY LEVEL CLASSIFICATIONS FROM AN INTERNATIONAL PHYSICAL ACTIVITY QUESTIONNAIRE (IPAQ) ASSESSMENT

Category 1 (Inactive)	Not active enough to meet criteria for categories 2 or 3
Category 2 (Minimally Active)	$\geq$3 days of vigorous activity of $\geq$20 min/day **OR** $\geq$5 days of moderate activity or walking of $\geq$30 min/day **OR** $\geq$5 days of any combination of walking or moderate or vigorous activity achieving a minimum of 600 MET · min · week^{-1}
Category 3 (HEPA Active [health-enhancing physical activity])	Vigorous activity $\geq$3 days/week achieving at least 1,500 MET · min · wk^{-1} **OR** 7 days of any combination of walking or moderate or vigorous activity achieving a minimum of 3,000 MET · min · wk^{-1}

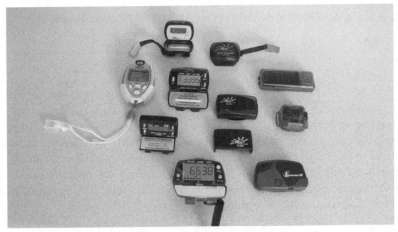

FIGURE 3.8. Many different models of pedometers and accelerometers are available to objectively measure physical activity.

with an objective assessment tool, a minimum period of observation is needed. Assessing physical activity for a minimum of 3 weekdays and at least 1 weekend day is optimal. For this purpose, many assessment approaches will involve a 1-week monitoring period.

INTERPRETATION

There can be numerous outcomes after assessing an individual's physical activity level, and this often depends on the assessment method chosen. For instance, some activity questionnaires may output calories expended; others will output an index range of 1–4, 1 being low active and 4 being the most active. Accelerometers may output the number of minutes a person spends in light-, moderate-, or vigorous-intensity activity on a daily basis, whereas a pedometer/step counter will yield the total number of steps taken on a particular day. Many of these output units are not interchangeable, or they become less valid in conversion. For instance, an attempt to convert steps accumulated per day into calories expended per day will result in the loss of some measurement accuracy. The validity of the method chosen and the selected output variable should always be considered when measuring physical activity levels.

TABLE 3.5. COMPARISON OF OBJECTIVE AND SUBJECTIVE PHYSICAL ACTIVITY ASSESSMENT TOOLS

	OBJECTIVE ASSESSMENT	SUBJECTIVE ASSESSMENT
Advantages	Concurrent measure of activity— as one moves it measures and records it Able to continuously record data for multiple days and weeks at a time Has an internal time clock, so activity can be time-stamped to a specific time of day	Inexpensive Population specific Can be administered to a large population
Disadvantages	Expensive Unable to assess type of activity (e.g., weight lifting, running up a hill, cycling into the wind)	Reliant on self-report and self-perception Memory dependent Poor in assessing typical activities of daily living (i.e., lifestyle activities)

TABLE 3.6. CLASSIFICATION OF PHYSICAL ACTIVITY BEHAVIOR

Sedentary/inactive	No moderate or vigorous activity
Insufficiently active	Some moderate or vigorous activity
Active	30 min of moderate activity ≥5 days per week and/or 20 min of vigorous activity 3 days per week or a combination of the two

Interpreting an individual's physical activity level can establish a profile of behavior, and classify the person as either engaging in enough activity to be health enhancing or engaging in so little activity as to warrant a classification of sedentary or inactive. Seasonal variation is also evident in physical activity behavior and needs to be considered when assessing and comparing physical activity patterns. Table 3.6 presents a classification system of physical activity behavior.

OTHER DISEASES AND CONDITIONS

There are other health-related issues that can easily be included in a screening, particularly if the program is a comprehensive health-based program. Although these issues related to the health-related physical fitness (HRPF) assessment are less common, some fitness professionals will offer these services.

PULMONARY DISEASE

There are many types of pulmonary (lung) diseases, some of which can manifest early in life (e.g., asthma). The *GETP8* notes that among the list of indications for pulmonary function testing are:

- to evaluate all smokers over the age of 45 years
- to assess health status before beginning strenuous physical activity programs
- to evaluate symptoms (e.g., dyspnea [shortness of breath], chronic cough, wheezing, or excessive mucus production)

Because some HRPF assessments require vigorous to maximal exertion, identifying those with abnormal pulmonary function would be valuable. Testing of pulmonary function can involve many different tests with specialized equipment that need to be administered by professionals with training in these procedures. However, there is a basic test that can be administered in screening programs that requires little equipment and can be conducted at a reasonable cost. The test requires the client to perform a maximal inhalation, followed by maximally exhaling as rapidly as possible. The total amount of air expelled in this procedure is called the forced vital capacity (FVC). The equipment used to measure the FVC will also measure the amount of air expelled in the first second of the procedure. This volume of air is called the forced expiratory volume in 1 second (FEV_1). It is common to use the ratio of these two variables, FEV_1/FVC, as the primary screening measure, with any value below 70% considered below normal limits. The interpretation can become more detailed as noted in Table 3.7. Those interested in more detailed interpretations should review the section on pulmonary function testing in Chapter 3 of the *GETP8*.

OSTEOPOROSIS

Osteoporosis is a disease that is characterized by low bone mass, which is often accompanied by bone fractures. Although often thought of as a condition seen primarily in

TABLE 3.7. INDICATIONS FOR SPIROMETRY

A. INDICATIONS FOR SPIROMETRY

Diagnosis
To evaluate symptoms, signs, or abnormal laboratory tests
To measure the effect of disease on pulmonary function
To screen individuals at risk of having pulmonary disease
To assess preoperative risk
To assess prognosis
To assess health status before beginning strenuous physical activity programs

Monitoring
To assess therapeutic intervention
To describe the course of diseases that affect lung function
To monitor people exposed to injurious agents
To monitor for adverse reactions to drugs with known pulmonary toxicity

Disability/Impairment Evaluations
To assess patients as part of a rehabilitation program
To assess risks as part of an insurance evaluation
To assess individuals for legal reasons

Public Health
Epidemiologic surveys
Derivation of reference equations
Clinical research

B. THE GLOBAL INITIATIVE FOR CHRONIC OBSTRUCTIVE LUNG DISEASE SPIROMETRIC CLASSIFICATION OF COPD SEVERITY BASED ON POSTBRONCHODILATOR FEV_1

Stage I	Mild	$FEV_1/FVC < 0.70$
		$FEV_1 \geq 80\%$ of predicted
Stage II	Moderate	$FEV_1/FVC < 0.70$
		$50\% \leq FEV_1 < 80\%$ predicted
Stage III	Severe	$FEV_1/FVC < 0.70$
		$30\% \leq FEV_1 < 50\%$ predicted
Stage IV	Very severe	$FEV_1/FVC < 0.70$
		$FEV_1 < 30\%$ predicted or $FEV_1 < 50\%$
		predicted plus chronic respiratory failure

C. THE AMERICAN THORACIC SOCIETY AND EUROPEAN RESPIRATORY SOCIETY CLASSIFICATION OF SEVERITY OF ANY SPIROMETRIC ABNORMALITY BASED ON FEV_1

Degree of Severity	FEV_1 % Predicted
Mild	Less than the LLN but ≥ 70
Moderate	60–69
Moderately severe	50–59
Severe	35–49
Very severe	<35

COPD, chronic obstructive pulmonary disease; FEV_1, forced expiratory volume in one second; FVC, forced vital capacity; respiratory failure, arterial partial pressure of oxygen (PaO_2) <8.0 kPa (60 mmHg) with or without arterial partial pressure of CO_2 (PaO_2) >6.7 kPa (50 mmHg) while breathing air at sea level; LLN, lower limit of normal.

Adapted from American College of Sports Medicine. *ACSM's Guidelines for Exercise Testing and Prescription*, 8th ed. Philadelphia (PA): Wolters Kluwer Health Ltd: 2009, 52 p.

Modified from Pauwels RA, Buist AS, Calverly PM, et al. Global strategy for the diagnosis, management, and prevention of chronic obstructive pulmonary disease. NHLBI/WHO Global Initiative for Chronic Obstructive Lung Disease (GOLD) Workshop summary. *Am J Respir Crit Care Med*. 2001;163:1256–76. Available from: http//www.goldcopd.com (last major revision, November 2006); Pellegrino R, Viegi G, Enright P, et al. Interpretive strategies for lung function tests. ATS/ERS Task Force: standardisation of lung function testing. *Eur Respir J*. 2005;26:948–68.

BOX 3.4	An Osteoporosis Screening Questionnaire

OSTEOPOROSIS: CAN IT HAPPEN TO YOU?

Osteoporosis is a major public health threat for 44 million Americans. Ten million individuals already have osteoporosis and 34 million more have low bone mass placing them at increased risk for developing osteoporosis and the fractures it causes. Eighty percent of those affected by osteoporosis are women. Known as "the silent thief," osteoporosis progresses without symptoms or pain until bones start to break, generally in the hip, spine, or wrist. Learn more about this bone-thinning disease that causes serious fractures.

Complete the questionnaire to determine your risk for developing osteoporosis.

	YES	NO
1. Do you have a small, thin frame and/or are you Caucasian or Asian?	☐	☐
2. Have you or a member of your immediate family broken a bone as an adult?	☐	☐
3. Are you a postmenopausal woman?	☐	☐
4. Have you had an early or surgically induced menopause?	☐	☐
5. Have you taken high doses of thyroid medication or used glucocorticoids (e.g., prednisone) for more than 3 months?	☐	☐
6. Have you taken, or are you taking, immunosuppressive medications or chemotherapy to treat cancer?	☐	☐
7. Is your diet low in dairy products and other sources of calcium?	☐	☐
8. Are you physically inactive?	☐	☐
9. Do you smoke cigarettes or drink alcohol in excess?	☐	☐

The more times you answer "yes," the greater your risk for developing osteoporosis. See your healthcare provider and contact the National Osteoporosis Foundation (NOF) for more information. Osteoporosis is a complex disease and not all of its causes are known. However, when certain risk factors are present, your likelihood of developing osteoporosis is increased. Therefore, it is important for you to determine your risk of developing osteoporosis and take action to prevent it now.

Osteoporosis is preventable if bone loss is detected early. If the questions suggest that you are at risk for developing osteoporosis, see your healthcare provider. Your healthcare provider may recommend that you have a bone mass measurement test. This test will safely and accurately measure your bone density and reliably predict your risk of future fracture.

If you already have osteoporosis, you can live actively and comfortably by seeking proper medical care and making some adjustments to your lifestyle. Your healthcare provider may prescribe a diet rich in calcium and vitamin D, a regular program of weight-bearing exercise, and medical treatment.

The NOF is the nation's leading authority for patients and healthcare providers seeking up-to-date, medically sound information and educational materials on the causes, prevention, detection, and treatment of osteoporosis. Please contact the NOF for more information on osteoporosis or to find out how you can join in the fight against this devastating disease.

National Osteoporosis Foundation. An osteoporosis screening questionnaire. From: *Osteoporosis: can it happen to you?* http://www.nof.org/prevention/risk_factor_questionnaire.pdf. Accessed February 21, 2009.

elderly women, the National Osteoporosis Foundation estimates that osteoporosis is a major health threat for 55% of Americans over age 50 years (10). The definitive test for diagnosing osteoporosis is a bone scan with a dual-energy x-ray absorptiometer, which is only available in clinical and research facilities. However, the fitness professional can administer a survey to help identify those who may be at greater risk. A version of a short, easy-to-administer and -interpret survey from the National Osteoporosis Foundation is shown in Box 3.4.

SUMMARY

Many fitness professionals can provide a valuable service by offering measurements of several different factors related to risk stratification assessment. These additional measurements do require specialized training and some instrumentation. Minimally, the fitness professional should know resources in the community where these services can be obtained and needs to be knowledgeable about the interpretation of the results from these risk factor assessments.

> > > **LABORATORY ACTIVITIES**

RESTING BLOOD PRESSURE ASSESSMENT

Data Collection
- Perform a calibration check of the aneroid manometer you will use for the laboratory. Record the results of this calibration check and provide an interpretation.
- Measure eight students' resting blood pressure and allow eight students to measure your resting blood pressure following the procedures in Box 3.2. Record the values that were measured on you below (do not let the technician see the previous measurement values).

Technician	#1	#2	#3	#4	#5	#6	#7	#8
Systolic BP								
Diastolic BP								

Written Report
1. Graph the data and comment on the variability in the measurements. Provide a critique of any deviations from recommended techniques you observed from watching the technicians. Using the mean values for systolic BP and diastolic BP, provide an interpretation of your resting blood pressure.
2. Provide responses for the following:
   - Describe the "white coat syndrome."
   - Explain how the principle of the auscultatory method is used for BP assessment.
   - Which of the Korotkoff sounds is used for systolic BP? What phase of the Korotkoff sounds is TRUE diastolic BP?

BODY MASS INDEX ASSESSMENT

Data Collection
- Perform any necessary calibration check of the equipment and report your findings.
- Measure eight students' height, weight, and waist circumference and allow eight students to make these measures on you following the procedures in this manual. Record the values that were measured on you below (do not let the technician see the previous measurement values). Calculate the BMI (show your work on these calculations).

Technician	#1	#2	#3	#4	#5	#6	#7	#8
Height								
Weight								
BMI								
Waist								

Written Report
1. Graph the data and comment on the variability in the measurements. Provide a critique of any deviations from recommended techniques you observed from watching the technicians.

2. Using the mean values for height, weight, and waist circumference, provide an interpretation of your BMI and disease risk.

INTERNATIONAL PHYSICAL ACTIVITY QUESTIONNAIRE ASSESSMENT

Data Collection
- Complete a short-form IPAQ. (Box 3.3).
- Ask two friends or relatives (one of each gender) who work full time to complete a short-form IPAQ.

Written Report
1. Perform the calculations of MET $\cdot$ min $\cdot$ week^{-1} on each of these three physical activity assessments.
2. Provide interpretations of each of the three subjects' IPAQ physical activity classifications and explain the criteria you used to choose the classification category.

> > > **CASE STUDY**

Jerome stopped by a booth that was a part of a health fair at the local mall. Jerome, who is 29 years old, had never had his cholesterol measured. He had a fingerstick blood sample taken, which was analyzed for total cholesterol and HDL cholesterol. The results reported that his total cholesterol was 287 mg $\cdot$ dL^{-1} and his HDL was 43 mg $\cdot$ dL^{-1}, and it was recommended that he have the test repeated again on another day. Jerome knew the ABC Fitness Center offered a service of performing lipid profiles, so he arranged to have a fasted blood test. The results from this test were total cholesterol 265 mg $\cdot$ dL^{-1}, HDL 38 mg $\cdot$ dL^{-1}, triglycerides 185 mg $\cdot$ dL^{-1}, LDL 190 mg $\cdot$ dL^{-1}, and glucose 106 mg $\cdot$ dL^{-1}. Provide an interpretation of these tests and explain what recommendation you would make to Jerome.

REFERENCES

1. American Diabetes Association. Standards of medical care in diabetes-2008. *Diabetes Care.* 2008;31: S12–33.
2. American Diabetes Association. Awareness of blood sugar critically lacking despite diabetes increase, American Diabetes Association survey finds. http://www.diabetes.org/for-media/2004-press-releases/ 03-23-04.jsp. 2004. Accessed July 24, 2008.
3. Chobanian AV, Bakis GL, Black HR, et al. The seventh report of the Joint National Committee on Prevention, Detection, Evaluation, and Treatment of High Blood Pressure. *JAMA.* 2003;289:2560–72.
4. Eckel RH, Krauss RM. American Heart Association call to action: obesity as a major risk factor for coronary heart disease. *Circulation.* 1998;86:340–44.
5. Haskell WL, Lee I-M, Pate RR, et al. Physical activity and public health: updated recommendation for adults. *Med Sci Sports Exerc.* 2007;39:1423–34.
6. International Physical Activity Questionnaire. Self-administered, short-form. May 2001. http://www.ipaq. ki.se/ipaq.htm. Accessed July 24, 2008.

7. National Cholesterol Education Program. Executive summary of the third report of the National Cholesterol Education Program (NCEP) expert panel on detection, evaluation, and treatment of high blood cholesterol in adults (Adult Treatment Panel III). *JAMA*. 2001;285:2486–97.

8. National Consumer League. New survey reveals consumers at risk of high cholesterol complications not taking steps to control it. http://www.nclnet.org/news/2004/cholesterol.htm. December 14, 2004. Accessed July 24, 2008.

9. National Institutes of Health, National Heart, Lung, and Blood Institute. *Clinical Guidelines on the Identification, Evaluation, and Treatment of Overweight and Obesity in Adults.* Bethesda (MD) June 1998. National Heart, Lung, and Blood Institute. NIH Pub. No. 98-4083.

10. National Osteoporosis Foundation. Fast facts on osteoporosis. http://www.nof.org/osteoporosis/diseasefacts.htm. Accessed February 21, 2009.

11. Pickering TG, Miller NH, Ogedegbe G, Krakoff LR, Artinina NT, Goff D. Call to action on the use and reimbursement for home blood pressure monitoring. A joint statement from the American Heart Association, American Society of Hypertension, and Preventative Cardiovascular Nurses Association. *Hypertension*. 2008;52:10–29.

12. Smith Jr SC, Allen J, Blair SN, et al. AHA/ACC Guidelines. AHA/ACC guidelines for secondary prevention for patients with coronary and atherosclerotic vascular disease: 2006 update. *Circulation*. 2006;113: 2363–72.

13. U.S. Department of Health and Human Services Physical Activity Guidelines for Americans. http://www.health.gov/paguidelines/ Washington, DC; 2008. Accessed February 21, 2009.

14. U.S. Department of Labor, Occupational Health and Safety Administration. Bloodborne pathogens regulations (Standards 29 CFR):1910.1030. http://www.osha.gov/pls/oshaweb/owadisp.show_document? p_ table=STANDARDS&p_id=10051. Accessed July 24, 2008.

Body Composition

WHY MEASURE BODY COMPOSITION?

In the most general sense, body composition is the study of the components of the body and their relative proportions. There is clinical value to knowing the amount of these varied body components. For example, the total amount (mass) and density of bone tissue is a critical measure to assess in the diagnosis and prognosis of osteoporosis. From a health-related physical fitness (HRPF) assessment point of view, body composition is defined as the relative proportions of fat and fat-free tissue in the body, typically expressed as a total body fat percentage. The focus of this chapter will be on the HRPF assessment of estimates of body fat percentage.

HEALTH IMPLICATIONS

In Chapters 2 and 3, the risks of obesity, as measured by body mass index (BMI) and waist circumference, were discussed. As a result of the high prevalence of obesity, many fitness professionals emphasize body composition assessment to their clients. However, the opposite end of the spectrum, low levels of body fat, also merits recognition. This is particularly relevant for girls and young women who are at greater risk for developing eating disorders and all athletes who are involved in sports where weight impacts performance. Unless clinically indicated, the assessment of body composition is typically not recommended for those with or at risk for developing an eating disorder.

It is also important to recognize changes in health-related components of body composition that accompany aging. Sarcopenia is defined as the age-related loss of muscle mass, with accompanying decreases in strength. Although assessment of the total amount of muscle mass is not obtained in the HRPF body composition assessment, it is a major component of the fat-free tissue that is estimated.

FUNCTIONAL IMPLICATIONS

Both obesity and sarcopenia result in some degree of functional impairment for individuals. Often, younger individuals are not as concerned about the accompanying health risks of conditions such as obesity and coronary heart disease, as they do not seem relevant to their daily lives. However, explaining and discussing the functional limitations of obesity may be a key in promoting an understanding of the negative effects of obesity. Such a discussion may encourage involvement in a fitness program.

Sarcopenia is increasingly being targeted as a major predictor of disability, resulting in nursing home institutionalization for older adults. Many adults perform only limited amounts of activities requiring high levels of muscular power, and most have neglected any forms of resistance exercise training. Thus, assessment of estimates of amount of muscle mass may be of value to older adults and actually motivate them to incorporate muscular fitness training into their exercise programs.

WHAT IS THE GOLD STANDARD TEST?

The simple, straightforward answer to the above question is that no method exists to accurately quantify the total amount of body fat in a living individual. Some clinical measures, as will be discussed in the next section, can provide accurate determinations of the amount of body fat in particular segments of the body. However, more investigations are needed prior to applying these expensive technologies in the determination of total body fat percentage.

4

Historically, the method of underwater (hydrostatic) weighing has been considered a gold standard for body fat percentage assessments. This method, which is used to determine body density, has typically been used as the standard against which other methods are compared. An overview of underwater weighing is provided later in this chapter.

CLINICAL MEASURES

Fitness professionals will have limited ability to obtain clinical measures of body composition for their clients. However, some clients may obtain these measures as part of their medical care and may bring the results to the fitness professional for advice.

MAGNETIC RESONANCE IMAGING AND COMPUTED TOMOGRAPHY

Magnetic resonance imaging (MRI) and computed tomography (CT) scans are typically used as diagnostic procedures for a variety of different diseases. These devices take a cross-sectional picture (think of this as one thin slice) of a region of the body. Recently, scientists have utilized these technologies to assess the change in amount of fat, bone, and muscle tissue related to different interventions, including exercise. Figure 4.1 shows an MRI scan of a segment of the thighs of a 30-year-old woman. Figure 4.2 shows a CT scan of a segment of the abdomen in an older man. Note the layer of subcutaneous fat on both of these scans. In these experimental research studies the scientists will take a scan at the same location before and after the intervention and then accurately measure the change in tissue at this segment of the body.

DUAL-ENERGY X-RAY ABSORPTIOMETRY

Dual-energy x-ray absorptiometry (DXA) measurements are ordered for individuals as a diagnostic test for osteoporosis. The main outcome measure from the DXA scan is bone density. However, as the x-ray technology has improved, it has allowed manufacturers

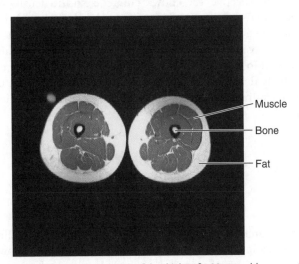

FIGURE 4.1. A magnetic resonance imaging scan of the thighs of a 30-year-old woman. Source: Ball State University—Dr. Todd Trappe.

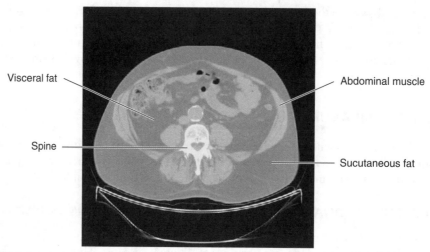

Visceral fat

Abdominal muscle

Spine

Sucutaneous fat

FIGURE 4.2. A computed tomography scan of the abdomen of an older man. Source: Ball State University—Dr. Todd Trappe.

to develop software to assess the relative amounts of other body components such as fat and lean tissue. Another valuable feature of DXA, CT, and MRI is that they allow the evaluation of regional body fat proportions. Figure 4.3 shows an example of one total body scan and the body composition report.

TESTS OF BODY VOLUME

The measurement of volume is used to determine density with the formula:

$$\text{Density} = \text{Mass} / \text{Volume}$$

Different types of body tissues have different density values. From an HRPF body composition assessment perspective, the known difference in the density of fat versus fat-free tissues is used to derive estimates of body fat percentage. Mass, or body weight, can be accurately determined following the procedures outlined in Chapter 3. Two widely used HRPF body composition assessment methods, underwater weighing and plethysmography, can be used to determine body volume. These methods are discussed below.

Once derived, body density (Db) is then used to estimate body fat percentage. Two commonly used generalized equations, shown below, are those developed by Siri (6) and Brozek et al. (2).

Siri equation:

$$\text{Body fat } (\%) = (495 / \text{Db}) - 450$$

Brozek equation:

$$\text{Body fat } (\%) = (457 / \text{Db}) - 414.2$$

However, as more research has been performed on individuals with different characteristics, population-specific equations have been developed and are shown in Table 4.1. These equations were developed around the knowledge that body mass can be differentiated on two components: fat mass (FM) and fat-free mass (FFM).

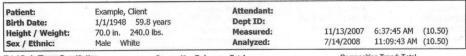

Ball State University
Human Performance Laboratory
Clinical Exercise Physiology Program

Patient:	Example, Client	**Attendant:**		
Birth Date:	1/1/1948 59.8 years	**Dept ID:**		
Height / Weight:	70.0 in. 240.0 lbs.	**Measured:**	11/13/2007 6:37:45 AM (10.50)	
Sex / Ethnic:	Male White	**Analyzed:**	7/14/2008 11:09:43 AM (10.50)	

Total Body Tissue Quantitation

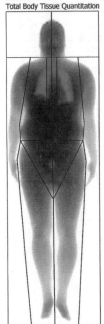

Composition Reference: Total

Tissue (%Fat)   Centile

40% 35% 30% 25% 20% 15% 10% 5% 0%   90 50 10 2

20 30 40 50 60 70 80 90 100
Age (years)

Composition Trend: Total

Fat (g)   Fat Free (g) [Gray]

37317 — 71164
37316 — 71163
37315 — 71162
37314 — 71161

58 59 60 61
Age (years)

Trend: Total

Measured Date	Age (years)	Tissue (%Fat)	Centile [2,3]	T.Mass (kg)	Region (%Fat)	Tissue (g)	Fat (g)	Lean (g)	BMC (g)	Fat Free (g)
11/13/2007	59.8	35.7	99	108.5	34.4	104,574	37,316	67,258	3,904	71,162

Trend: Fat Distribution

Measured Date	Age (years)	Android (%Fat)	Gynoid (%Fat)	A/G Ratio	Total Body (%Fat)
11/13/2007	59.8	46.1	34.2	1.35	35.7

COMMENTS:

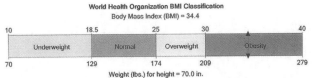

World Health Organization BMI Classification
Body Mass Index (BMI) = 34.4

10	18.5	25	30	40
Underweight	Normal	Overweight	Obesity	
70	129	174	209	279

Weight (lbs.) for height = 70.0 in.

Image not for diagnosis

Printed: 7/14/2008 11:10:13 AM (10.50)76:0.15:76.92:62.4 0.00:-1.00
4.80x13.00 16.5:%Fat=35.7%
0.00:0.00 0.00:0.00
Filename: hn2grj7vb.dfb
Scan Mode: Thick   0.8 µGy

2 -NHANES/USA Total Body Reference Population (v107)
3 -Matched for Age, Weight (males 25-100 kg), Ethnic

GE Healthcare

Lunar Prodigy
DF+10199

FIGURE 4.3. A body composition report from a total body dual-energy x-ray absorptiometry scan. Source: Ball State University—Clinical Exercise Physiology Program.

UNDERWATER (HYDROSTATIC) WEIGHING

The underwater weighing method is based on Archimedes' principle that states that a body immersed in a fluid is buoyed up by a force equal to the weight of the displaced fluid. This method measures body volume via water displacement. To determine body volume using the underwater weighing method requires measurements of body weight

Ball State University
Human Performance Laboratory
Clinical Exercise Physiology Program

Patient:	Example, Client	Attendant:		
Birth Date:	1/1/1948 59.8 years	Dept ID:		
Height / Weight:	70.0 in. 240.0 lbs.	Measured:	11/13/2007	6:37:45 AM (10.50)
Sex / Ethnic:	Male White	Analyzed:	7/14/2008	11:09:43 AM (10.50)

BODY COMPOSITION

Region	Tissue (%Fat)	Region (%Fat)	Tissue (g)	Fat (g)	Lean (g)	BMC (g)	Total Mass (kg)
Left Arm	26.0	24.8	5,264	1,371	3,893	260	-
Left Leg	31.8	30.4	15,430	4,904	10,526	714	-
Left Trunk	41.4	40.4	28,830	11,923	16,908	684	-
Left Total	35.6	34.4	52,680	18,780	33,900	1,981	-
Right Arm	26.0	24.9	5,314	1,383	3,931	252	-
Right Leg	31.8	30.5	15,511	4,935	10,575	688	-
Right Trunk	41.4	40.4	28,294	11,706	16,588	708	-
Right Total	35.7	34.4	51,894	18,536	33,358	1,923	-
Arms	26.0	24.8	10,578	2,754	7,824	512	-
Legs	31.8	30.4	30,941	9,839	21,102	1,402	-
Trunk	41.4	40.4	57,125	23,628	33,496	1,393	-
Android	46.1	45.7	10,249	4,720	5,529	84	-
Gynoid	34.2	33.3	15,827	5,414	10,413	416	-
Total	35.7	34.4	104,574	37,316	67,258	3,904	108.5

FAT MASS RATIOS

Trunk/ Total	Legs/ Total	(Arms+Legs)/ Trunk
0.63	0.26	0.53

3 -Matched for Age, Weight (males 25-100 kg), Ethnic

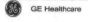 GE Healthcare

Lunar Prodigy
DF+10199

FIGURE 4.3. (*Continued*)

before entering the water and the loss of body weight when submerged underwater. The underwater weight is influenced by two amounts of air trapped in the body, residual lung volume and gas in the gastrointestinal (GI) system. This trapped air contributes to buoyancy and thus needs to be factored into the calculation of underwater weight. Ideally, residual volume should be measured; however, it is often predicted, and a constant

TABLE 4.1. FORMULAS FOR CONVERSION OF BODY DENSITY (Db) TO PERCENT BODY FAT

POPULATION	AGE	SEX	% BODY FAT[a]
Race			
American Indian	18–60	Female	(4.81/Db)–4.34
Black	18–32	Male	(4.37/Db)–3.93
	24–79	Female	(4.85/Db)–4.39
Hispanic	20–40	Female	(4.87/Db)–4.41
Japanese Native	18–48	Male	(4.97/Db)–4.52
		Female	(4.76/Db)–4.28
	61–78	Male	(4.87/Db)–4.41
		Female	(4.95/Db)–4.50
White	7–12	Male	(5.30/Db)–4.89
		Female	(5.35/Db)–4.95
	13–16	Male	(5.07/Db)–4.64
		Female	(5.10/Db)–4.66
	17–19	Male	(4.99/Db)–4.55
		Female	(5.05/Db)–4.62
	20–80	Male	(4.95/Db)–4.50
		Female	(5.01/Db)–4.57
Levels of body fatness			
Anorexia	15–30	Female	(5.26/Db)–4.83
Obese	17–62	Male	(5.00/Db)–4.56

[a]Percent body fat is obtained by multiplying the value calculated from the equation by 100.

American College of Sports Medicine. *ACSM's Guidelines for Exercise Testing and Prescription*, 8th ed. Philadelphia (PA): Wolters Kluwer Health Ltd: 2009, 70 p.

Adapted from Heyward VH, Stolarczyk LM. Body Composition Assessment. Champaign (IL): *Human Kinetics*; 1996. p12.

value of 100 mL is used for GI gas. Common formulas used to estimate residual volume based on gender, height (cm), and age are:

Men: Residual volume (L) = [0.019 · Height (cm)] + [0.0155 · Age (years)] − 2.24 (1)

Women: Residual volume (L): [0.032 · Height (cm)] + [0.009 · Age (years)] − 3.90 (4)

Also, because the density of the water varies with temperature, the temperature of the water needs to be measured. The density of water can be determined at the following web site: http://www.simetric.co.uk/si_water.htm#tenth (Accessed February 21, 2009).

Typically a freestanding tank of water is used for the underwater weighing procedure, which includes a chair for the client, attached to a scale for weight measurement as shown in Figure 4.4. The assessment procedures for underwater weighing are provided in Box 4.1. Owing to the effort requirement to maximally exhale while being submerged underwater, the results of this test are dependent on the client's effort and success in performing the technique correctly. The formula for calculating body volume from this procedure is:

Body volume = ({[Body weight (g) − Underwater weight (g)] / Water density}
    − [Residual volume (mL) + 100 mL])

Finally, body weight is divided by body volume to derive Db.

PLETHYSMOGRAPHY

A body plethysmograph can determine changes in volume (V) with measures of pressure (P) according to Boyle's Law (P1V1 = P2V2, if temperature is constant). There is

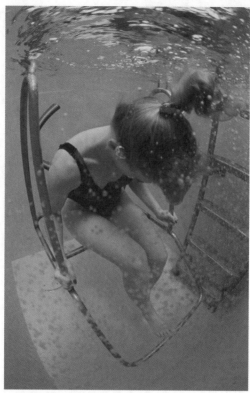

FIGURE 4.4. The underwater weighing procedure.

at least one manufacturer that sells a whole body plethysmograph to provide measures of body volume by assessing air displacement. This plethysmograph has two chambers. Measurements of pressure and volume are first made with the front chamber empty, then with a standard cylinder of known volume to calibrate the system, and then finally with a person in the front chamber. The procedure requires the client to follow similar pretest standardizations as for underwater weighing (see Box 4.1). Additionally, the client must wear only tight-fitting clothing made of nylon (typically a swimsuit or cycling shorts and a jog bra) and a swim cap to control for temperature variations caused by hair on the head as shown in Figure 4.5. The client only needs to sit still while the instrument makes the measures of body volume, thus eliminating the performance requirements of underwater weighing, which makes it an easier and less time-consuming procedure. The outcome measure of body volume is then used to calculate Db.

ANTHROPOMETRY

Anthropometry is the measurement of the human body, which includes measures of circumferences or girths, as well as skinfolds. Anthropometric measurements are made at a variety of specific sites on the body.

SKINFOLD MEASUREMENTS

Skinfold measurements can be used to estimate body fat percentage based on the assumption that the amount of subcutaneous fat in a particular skinfold is proportional to

BOX 4.1	**Procedures for Underwater Weighing**

PRETEST STANDARDIZATIONS

1. Clients should be in a normally hydrated state and should not have eaten for at least 3 hours.
2. Immediately prior to the assessment clients should empty their bladder and attempt to empty their bowels.
3. Clients should remove any makeup, body oils, and jewelry prior to entering the water.
4. Clients should wear a tight-fitting swimsuit to eliminate air trapping.
5. Explain to clients that they should begin exhaling as they gently submerge themselves under the water and to continue exhaling as much as possible. At that point they need to remain underwater as long as possible and remain as still as possible to obtain a stable underwater weight reading. This procedure will need to be repeated multiple times (typically 5–10) as there is generally a learning effect for this procedure.

ASSESSMENT PROCEDURES

1. Obtain a body weight measurement on clients before they enter the water.
2. Measure the temperature of the water.
3. Have clients enter the water and sit on the suspended chair.
4. Have clients submerge themselves underwater, following the instructions provided. Note: Some clients may require that the chair be weighted if while performing the procedure a part of their body breaks the surface of the water (because of buoyancy).
5. Repeat step 4 until at least three consecutive underwater weight readings do not increase.

the total amount of overall body fat. At first glance, pinching a fold of skin and applying a set of calipers to measure the distance appears to be a simple skill. However, consistently obtaining accurate skinfold measurements requires a good-quality skinfold caliper, specific training, and a significant amount of practice.

The skinfold caliper should deliver a specific amount of force, and good-quality calipers come with this assurance from the manufacturer. One source of variability in skinfold measurements occurs from using a caliper that does not deliver the recommended amount of force. Ideally, this level of force should be checked periodically. The caliper distance measurement should also be checked using a simple standardized calibrations block as shown in Figure 4.6.

The skinfold procedure requires that the technician grasp the skin with the thumb and index finger approximately 3 inches (7.5 cm) apart and firmly pull the skin, with the underlying subcutaneous fat, away from the limb or torso. The fold will contain two layers of skin with only fat in between. If there is any doubt about the fold containing some muscle tissue, the client should be instructed to contract the muscle at that site to allow the technician to feel whether any muscle is in the fold. The arms of the caliper are opened and applied to the skinfold by gradually releasing the pressure on the caliper arms. Note that the measurement scale should be facing up for viewing, which for most calipers

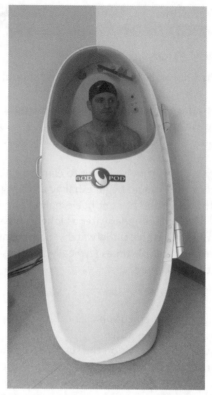

FIGURE 4.5. A client having his body fat percentage estimated using whole body plethysmography.

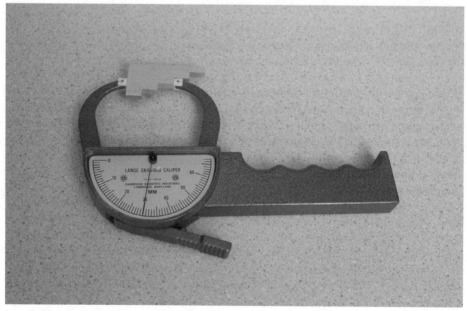

FIGURE 4.6. The method to check the distance calibration of a pair of skinfold calipers.

requires a right-handed grip. Box 4.2 provides descriptions of the standardized skinfold sites along with procedural recommendations as shown in Figure 4.7A–G. Careful attention to the anatomic landmarks and the actual measurement of distances is important for obtaining accurate and reliable measures. Once the location is identified, it should be marked on

BOX 4.2	Descriptions of the Standardized Skinfold Sites Along with Procedural Recommendations

SKINFOLD SITE

Abdominal	Vertical fold; 2 cm to the right side of the umbilicus
Triceps	Vertical fold; on the posterior midline of the upper arm, halfway between the acromion and olecranon processes, with the arm held freely to the side of the body
Biceps	Vertical fold; on the anterior aspect of the arm over the belly of the biceps muscle, 1 cm above the level used to mark the triceps site
Chest/pectoral	Diagonal fold; one half the distance between the anterior axillary line and the nipple (men), or one third of the distance between the anterior axillary line and the nipple (women)
Medial calf	Vertical fold; at the maximum circumference of the calf on the midline of its medial border
Midaxillary	Vertical fold; on the midaxillary line at the level of the xiphoid process of the sternum (An alternate method is a horizontal fold taken at the level of the xiphoid/sternal border in the midaxillary line.)
Subscapular	Diagonal fold (at a 45-degree angle); 1 to 2 cm below the inferior angle of the scapula
Suprailiac	Diagonal fold; in line with the natural angle of the iliac crest taken in the anterior axillary line immediately superior to the iliac crest
Thigh	Vertical fold; on the anterior midline of the thigh, midway between the proximal border of the patella and the inguinal crease (hip)

PROCEDURES

- All measurements should be made on the right side of the body with the subject standing upright.
- The caliper should be placed directly on the skin surface, 1 cm away from the thumb and finger, perpendicular to the skinfold, and halfway between the crest and the base of the fold.
- A pinch should be maintained while reading the caliper.
- Wait 1 to 2 seconds (not longer) before reading caliper.
- Take duplicate measures at each site, and retest if duplicate measurements are not within 1 to 2 mm.
- Rotate through measurement sites, or allow time for skin to regain normal texture and thickness.

Adapted from American College of Sports Medicine. *ACSM's Guidelines for Exercise Testing and Prescription*, 8th ed. Philadelphia (PA): Wolters Kluwer Health Ltd: 2009, 67 p.

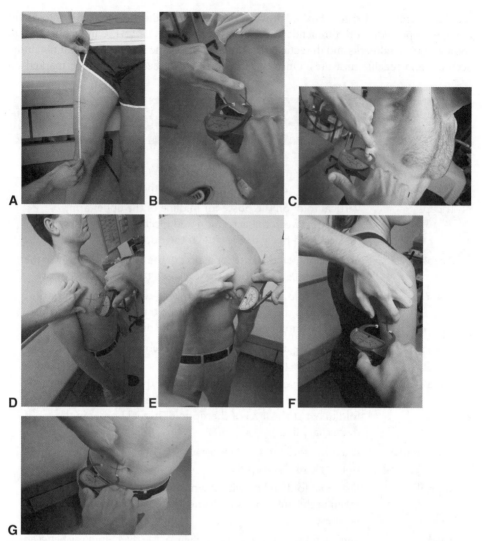

FIGURE 4.7. A: The thigh skinfold site. **B:** The suprailiac skinfold site. **C:** The midaxillary skinfold site. **D:** The chest skinfold site. **E:** The subscapular skinfold site. **F:** The triceps skinfold site. **G:** The abdomen skinfold site.

the skin with a water-solvent ink pen. Variation in the location of the skinfold site and the application of the calipers are the two largest sources of error in skinfold measures. Figure 4.8A, B illustrates examples of correct and incorrect procedures for skinfold assessments.

Because the proportion of subcutaneous to total fat is known to vary between genders, between ethnic groups, and with age, different prediction equations have been developed to estimate body fat percentage. There are also generalized equations that can be used for most clients as well as specialized population-specific equations that can be used if working with a homogeneous group of people (e.g., female collegiate volleyball players). The most commonly used method for estimating Db via skinfold measurement employs the generalized equations provided in Box 4.3. For both men and women, there are three options, one that uses seven and two that use three different skinfold sites (3,5). Theoretically, the more skinfold sites measured, the better is the prediction

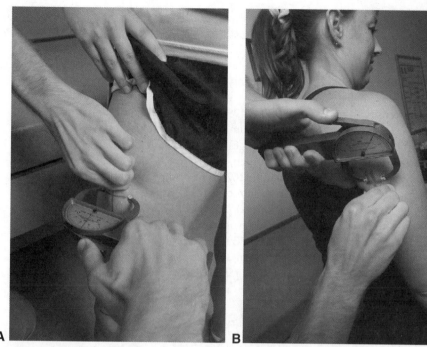

FIGURE 4.8. A: Example of correct procedures for skinfold assessments. **B:** Example of incorrect procedures for skinfold assessments.

of body fat. However, for most clients there are small differences between the three- and seven-site methods, so the three-site methods are typically used.

CIRCUMFERENCES MEASUREMENTS

Circumference measurements have the advantages of being easily learned, quickly conducted, and inexpensively administered. The only equipment requirement is an inexpensive measurement tape. Circumferences, also known as girths, are best used to measure changes in size of a body part. Perhaps the most important application is the use of circumferences to determine body fat distribution as was covered in Chapter 3. Circumferences can also be used to measure muscle girth size and therefore quantify changes in muscle with specific training (e.g., resistance weight training) or to help monitor sarcopenia.

There are some equations that use either circumferences or a combination of circumference and skinfold measurements to estimate body fat percentage. However, this approach is not commonly used. Box 4.4 provides descriptions of the standardized circumference sites along with procedural recommendations.

BIOELECTRICAL IMPEDANCE ANALYSIS

One other method for estimating body fat percentage that has gained popularity in commercial fitness programs is bioelectrical impedance analysis (BIA). The bioelectrical impedance analyzer introduces a small electrical current into the body and measures the resistance to that current as it passes through the body. Current will flow more readily through body water, which contains electrolytes. Fat contains only small amounts of water so current will not flow easily (i.e., impeded) through areas containing fat. Conversely,

---

BOX 4.3	Generalized Skinfold Equations

MEN

- **Seven-Site Formula** (chest, midaxillary, triceps, subscapular, abdomen, suprailiac, thigh)

  Body density = $1.112 - 0.00043499$ (sum of seven skinfolds)
  $+ 0.00000055$ (sum of seven skinfolds)^2
  $- 0.00028826$ (age) *[SEE 0.008 or ~3.5% fat]*

- **Three-Site Formula** (chest, abdomen, thigh)

  Body density = $1.10938 - 0.0008267$ (sum of three skinfolds)
  $+ 0.0000016$ (sum of three skinfolds)^2
  $- 0.0002574$ (age) *[SEE 0.008 or ~3.4% fat]*

- **Three-Site Formula** (chest, triceps, subscapular)

  Body density = $1.1125025 - 0.0013125$ (sum of three skinfolds)
  $+ 0.0000055$ (sum of three skinfolds)^2
  $- 0.000244$ (age) *[SEE 0.008 or ~3.6% fat]*

WOMEN

- **Seven-Site Formula** (chest, midaxillary, triceps, subscapular, abdomen, suprailiac, thigh)

  Body density = $1.097 - 0.00046971$ (sum of seven skinfolds)
  $+ 0.00000056$ (sum of seven skinfolds)^2
  $- 0.00012828$ (age) *[SEE 0.008 or ~3.8% fat]*

- **Three-Site Formula** (triceps, suprailiac, thigh)

  Body density = $1.099421 - 0.0009929$ (sum of three skinfolds)
  $+ 0.0000023$ (sum of three skinfolds)^2
  $- 0.0001392$ (age) *[SEE 0.009 or ~3.9% fat]*

- **Three-Site Formula** (triceps, suprailiac, abdominal)

  Body density = $1.089733 - 0.0009245$ (sum of three skinfolds)
  $+ 0.0000025$ (sum of three skinfolds)^2
  $- 0.0000979$ (age) *[SEE 0.009 or ~3.9% fat]*

American College of Sports Medicine. *ACSM's Guidelines for Exercise Testing and Prescription*, 8th ed. Philadelphia (PA): Wolters Kluwer Health Ltd: 2009, 68 p.

Adapted from Jackson AS, Pollock ML. Practical assessment of body composition. *Phys Sport Med.* 1985;13:76–90. Pollock ML, Schmidt DH, Jackson AS. Measurement of cardiorespiratory fitness and body composition in the clinical setting. *Comp Ther.* 1980;6:12–7.

---

lean tissue, which contains large amounts of water, and thus electrolytes, will be a good electrical conductor.

Because the BIA measure is dependent on the total body water and is based on assumptions about water content of fat and lean tissues, anything that changes a person's hydration status will affect the prediction of body fat percentage. Patients who are prescribed a medication that has a diuretic property should avoid this test, as the results will probably not be valid. To control for factors that affect hydration status, the following pretest conditions should be used prior to a BIA measurement:

- No alcohol consumption for the previous 48 hours before the test
- No products with diuretic properties (e.g., caffeine, chocolate) for the previous 24 hours before the test

BOX 4.4	**Standardized Description of Circumference Sites and Procedures**

Abdomen: With the subject standing upright and relaxed, a horizontal measure is taken at the greatest anterior extension of the abdomen, usually at the level of the umbilicus.

Arm: With the subject standing erect and arms hanging freely at the sides with hands facing the thigh, a horizontal measure is taken midway between the acromion and olecranon processes.

Buttocks/hips: With the subject standing erect and feet together, a horizontal measure is taken at the maximal circumference of buttocks. This measure is used for the hip measure in a waist/hip measure.

Calf: With the subject standing erect (feet apart ~20 cm), a horizontal measure is taken at the level of the maximum circumference between the knee and the ankle, perpendicular to the long axis.

Forearm: With the subject standing, arms hanging downward but slightly away from the trunk and palms facing anteriorly, a measure perpendicular to the long axis at the maximal circumference.

Hips/thigh: With the subject standing, legs slightly apart (~10 cm), a horizontal measure is taken at the maximal circumference of the hip/proximal thigh, just below the gluteal fold.

Midthigh: With the subject standing and one foot on a bench so the knee is flexed at 90 degrees, a measure is taken midway between the inguinal crease and the proximal border of the patella, perpendicular to the long axis.

Waist: With the subject standing, arms at the sides, feet together, and abdomen relaxed, a horizontal measure is taken at the narrowest part of the torso (above the umbilicus and below the xiphoid process). The National Obesity Task Force (NOTF) suggests obtaining a horizontal measure directly above the iliac crest as a method to enhance standardization. Unfortunately, current formulae are not predicated on the NOTF suggested site.

PROCEDURES

- All measurements should be made with a flexible yet inelastic tape measure.
- The tape should be placed on the skin surface without compressing the subcutaneous adipose tissue.
- If a Gulick spring-loaded handle is used, the handle should be extended to the same marking with each trial.
- Take duplicate measures at each site, and retest if duplicate measurements are not within 5 mm.
- Rotate through measurement sites or allow time for skin to regain normal texture.

Adapted from American College of Sports Medicine. *ACSM's Guidelines for Exercise Testing and Prescription,* 8th ed. Philadelphia (PA): Wolters Kluwer Health Ltd: 2009, 65–66 p.

Modified from Callaway CW, Chumlea WC, Bouchard C. Circumferences. In: Lohman TG, Roche AF, Martorell R, editors. *Anthropometric Standardization Reference Manual.* Champaign (IL): Human Kinetics; 1988;39–54.

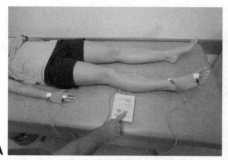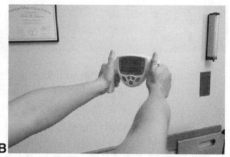

A **B**

FIGURE 4.9. A: A bioelectrical impedance analysis (BIA) device that utilizes electrodes on the hand and foot. **B:** A handheld BIA device.

- No exercise for the previous 12 hours before the test
- No eating or drinking for the previous 4 hours before the test
- Void bladder completely within 30 minutes of the test

The procedures for BIA measurement are specific to the actual BIA device that is being utilized as shown in Figure 4.9A, B. Calibration of most devices is limited to an internal system

TABLE 4.2. BODY FAT NORMS—MEN

			AGE				
%	20–29	30–39	40–49	50–59	60–69	70–79	
99	4.2	7.0	9.2	10.9	11.5	13.6	
95	6.3	9.9	12.8	14.4	15.5	15.2	VL[a]
90	7.9	11.9	14.9	16.7	17.6	17.8	
85	9.2	13.3	16.3	18.0	18.8	19.2	
80	10.5	14.5	17.4	19.1	19.7	20.4	E
75	11.5	15.5	18.4	19.9	20.6	21.1	
70	12.7	16.5	19.1	20.7	21.3	21.6	
65	13.9	17.4	19.9	21.3	22.0	22.5	
60	14.8	18.2	20.6	22.1	22.6	23.1	G
55	15.8	19.0	21.3	22.7	23.2	23.7	
50	16.6	19.7	21.9	23.2	23.7	24.1	
45	17.4	20.4	22.6	23.9	24.4	24.4	
40	18.6	21.3	23.4	24.6	25.2	24.8	F
35	19.6	22.1	24.1	25.3	26.0	25.4	
30	20.6	23.0	24.8	26.0	26.7	26.0	
25	21.9	23.9	25.7	26.8	27.5	26.7	
20	23.1	24.9	26.6	27.8	28.4	27.6	P
15	24.6	26.2	27.7	28.9	29.4	28.9	
10	26.3	27.8	29.2	30.3	30.9	30.4	
5	28.9	30.2	31.2	32.5	32.9	32.4	
1	33.3	34.3	35.0	36.4	36.8	35.5	VP
n =	1826	8373	10442	6079	1836	301	

Total n = 28,857
Norms are based on Cooper Clinic patients.

[a]Very Lean—No less than 3% body fat is recommended for males.

VL, very lean; E, excellent; G, good; F, fair; P, poor; VP, very poor.

American College of Sports Medicine. *ACSM's Guidelines for Exercise Testing and Prescription*, 8th ed. Philadelphia, (PA): Wolters Kluwer Health Ltd: 2009, 71 p.

The Cooper Institute for Aerobics Research. *Physical Fitness Assessments and Norms for Adults and Law Enforcement*, 2002. Available online at http://www.cooperinstitute.org, with permission.

check. Some devices require placing electrodes on the hand and foot to collect the information. Others require that a person hold handles or stand on a platform to gather the information. There are no specific procedural requirements for the clients. Prior to the measurement, demographic data including age, gender, height, and weight are entered. Ideally, the client should have height and weight measured according to the procedures outlined in Chapter 3. Some of the BIA devices may also allow input of some category of physical activity status as well as ethnic/racial group. Similar to the skinfold method, BIA estimates of body fat percentage can be made from either generalized or population-specific equations and some BIA devices allow the user to select an equation. Generally, most devices do not report the actual impedance values, so the raw data are unavailable for use in other equations.

INTERPRETATION

Normative standards for body fat percentage have not been developed in part because of the differences in measures between the various methods and variable standard errors of estimate (SEEs) for these methods. The American College of Sports Medicine (ACSM) has used the reference values established by the Cooper Institute, shown in Tables 4.2 and 4.3,

TABLE 4.3. BODY FAT NORMS—WOMEN

			AGE				
%	20–29	30–39	40–49	50–59	60–69	70–79	
99	9.8	11.0	12.6	14.6	13.9	14.6	
95	13.6	14.0	15.6	17.2	17.7	16.6	VL[a]
90	14.8	15.6	17.2	19.4	19.8	20.3	
85	15.8	16.6	18.6	20.9	21.4	23.0	
80	16.5	17.4	19.8	22.5	23.2	24.0	E
75	17.3	18.2	20.8	23.8	24.8	25.0	
70	18.0	19.1	21.9	25.1	25.9	26.2	
65	18.7	20.0	22.8	26.0	27.0	27.7	
60	19.4	20.8	23.8	27.0	27.9	28.6	G
55	20.1	21.7	24.8	27.9	28.7	29.7	
50	21.0	22.6	25.6	28.8	29.8	30.4	
45	21.9	23.5	26.5	29.7	30.6	31.3	
40	22.7	24.6	27.6	30.4	31.3	31.8	F
35	23.6	25.6	28.5	31.4	32.5	32.7	
30	24.5	26.7	29.6	32.5	33.3	33.9	
25	25.9	27.7	30.7	33.4	34.3	35.3	
20	27.1	29.1	31.9	34.5	35.4	36.0	P
15	28.9	30.9	33.5	35.6	36.2	37.4	
10	31.4	33.0	35.4	36.7	37.3	38.2	
5	35.2	35.8	37.4	38.3	39.0	39.3	
1	38.9	39.4	39.8	40.4	40.8	40.5	VP
n =	1360	3597	3808	2366	849	136	

Total n = 12,116

Norms are based on Cooper Clinic patients.

[a]Very Lean—No less than 10–13% body fat is recommended for females.

VL, very lean; E, excellent; G, good; F, fair; P, poor; VP, very poor.

American College of Sports Medicine. *ACSM's Guidelines for Exercise Testing and Prescription*, 8th ed. Philadelphia, (PA): Wolters Kluwer Health Ltd: 2009, 72 p.

The Cooper Institute for Aerobics Research. *Physical Fitness Assessments and Norms for Adults and Law Enforcement*, 2002. Available online at http://www.cooperinstitute.org, with permission.

TABLE 4.4. STANDARD ERROR OF ESTIMATE FOR DIFFERENT BODY FAT ASSESSMENT METHODS

METHOD FOR ESTIMATING BODY FAT PERCENTAGE	STANDARD ERROR OF ESTIMATE
Air displacement (BOD POD)	±2.2% to ±3.7%
Bioelectrical impedance analysis	±3.5% to ±5%
Dual-energy x-ray absorptiometry	±1.8%
Skinfold measurements	±3.5%
Underwater weighing	±2.5%

Adapted from American College of Sports Medicine. *ACSM's Resource Manual for Guidelines for Exercise Testing and Prescription*, 6th ed. Philadelphia (PA): Wolters Kluwer Health Ltd: 2009, 277 p.

for interpretation. It is important to recognize that these values are based on the population that has received these measures and are expressed as percentiles, which may limit their usefulness.

As discussed in Chapter 1, whenever an assessment is based on estimation, the interpretation should include an expression of the SEE. Table 4.4 provides the SEE values for hydrostatic weighing, plethysmography, skinfolds, and BIA.

ESTIMATION OF GOAL BODY WEIGHT

For those individuals who desire to change body composition, it is helpful to provide them with an estimation of body weight at a goal body fat percentage. A simple method to derive an estimate of a goal body weight is based on the following equation.

$$\text{Goal body weight} = \text{Fat-free weight} / (1 - [\text{Goal \% body fat} / 100])$$

An example of the calculation of goal body weight for a man who weighs 200 pounds with an estimated body fat of 25% and a goal body fat of 15% is as follows:

Determine fat-free weight:

$$\text{Fat-free weight} = \text{Body weight} \cdot ([100 - \% \text{ Body fat}] / 100)$$
$$= 200 \cdot ([100 - 25] / 100) = 150 \text{ lbs}$$

Determine goal body weight:

$$\text{Goal body weight} = 150 / (1 - [15 / 100])$$
$$= 176.4 \text{ lbs}$$

SUMMARY

Body composition measurements are performed as part of an HRPF evaluation and also provide important information related to functional status. Although there is not a true gold standard measure of body composition, there are many methods that can provide helpful information.

SKINFOLD ESTIMATION OF BODY FAT PERCENTAGE

Data Collection

Work in groups of three and make all skinfold measurements on every member of your group (one technician, one subject, one recorder). Use Box 4.2 as a guide for identifying appropriate skinfold sites. Take each measurement twice (take a third if the first two differ by more than 2 mm) and average the two closest measures. Use Box 4.3 (to calculate body density from skinfold measurements) and use the Siri equation (6) to calculate % fat from body density (when using body density to calculate % body fat, carry the body density value out four places past the decimal). Calculate your body fat using the seven-site formula and EACH of the three-site formulas in Box 4.3. Show your calculations on a separate sheet of paper and hand them in with the rest of the assignment. Record values obtained on you.

Written Report

1. Using your % fat value for the seven-site formula for the first technician, what range of values would represent ±1 SEE unit encompassing 68% of the population with these same % fat values?
2. How did the % fat values obtained from the seven- and three-site formulas compare for the first technician?
3. How reliable were the two technicians in determining % body fat and the skinfold measures at each site?
4. Using the seven-site formula, what is your fat weight from each technician?
5. Using the seven-site formula, what is your fat-free weight from each technician?

Technician: _____ Height (in. or cm): _____ Weight (lbs or kg): _____

		Skinfolds			Mean
Abdominal	_____ mm	_____ mm	_____ mm	=	_____ mm
Triceps	_____ mm	_____ mm	_____ mm	=	_____ mm
Biceps	_____ mm	_____ mm	_____ mm	=	_____ mm
Chest/pectoral	_____ mm	_____ mm	_____ mm	=	_____ mm
Midaxillary	_____ mm	_____ mm	_____ mm	=	_____ mm
Subscapular	_____ mm	_____ mm	_____ mm	=	_____ mm
Suprailiac	_____ mm	_____ mm	_____ mm	=	_____ mm
Thigh	_____ mm	_____ mm	_____ mm	=	_____ mm

Seven-site formula: _____ % fat
Three-site formula: _____ % fat
Three-site formula: _____ % fat

> > > **CASE STUDY**

David is a 45-year-old man who came in to the ABC Fitness Club for a body composition evaluation. David weighed 187 pounds and was tested in a whole body plethysmograph. His body volume was determined to be 81.5 L. What is David's estimated body fat percentage, including the SEE? Provide David with an interpretation of his estimated body fat percentage using a percentile score. If David desired to be at the 75th percentile for men his age, what is his goal body weight at that desired level of body fat?

REFERENCES

1. Boren HG, Kory RC, Snyder JC. The Veteran's Administration Army Cooperative study of pulmonary function. II. The lung volume and its subdivisions in normal men. *Am J Med.* 1966;41:96–114.
2. Brozek J, Grade F, Anderson J. Densitometric analysis of body composition: revision of some quantitative assumptions. *Ann N Y Acad Sci.* 1963;110:113–40.
3. Jackson AS, Pollock ML. Practical assessment of body composition. *Phys Sport Med.* 1985;13:76–90.
4. O'Brien RJ, Drizd TA. Roentgenographic determination of total lung capacity: normal values from a national population survey. *Am Rev Respir Dis.* 1983;128:949–52.
5. Pollock ML, Schmidt DH, Jackson AS. Measurement of cardiorespiratory fitness and body composition in the clinical setting. *Comp Ther.* 1980;6:12–7.
6. Siri WE. The gross composition of the body. *Adv Biol Med Physiol.* 1956;4:239–280, 1956.

Muscular Fitness

5 CHAPTER

UNIQUE ASSESSMENT PRINCIPLES

Muscular strength and muscular endurance are measurable components of health-related physical fitness (HRPF). One unique aspect of muscle measurements is that there are approximately 700 skeletal muscles in the human body, each of which can yield a different level of performance. So, unlike body composition and cardiorespiratory endurance, there is no single measurement that provides an assessment of an individual's muscular strength or muscular endurance. Then, to further complicate the assessment of muscular fitness, there are different types of muscular contractions. Because many muscular contractions involve more than one muscle, performance can vary with technique and variation of the method employed to load the muscle. All these variable factors can influence muscular strength and muscular endurance assessments (1).

TYPES OF CONTRACTIONS

Basically, there are two principal types of muscular contractions: static and dynamic. During a static contraction, the muscle generates force without movement taking place. This may involve pushing or pulling against an immovable object or holding an object in place. These are also called isometric ("iso" meaning equal and metric meaning length) contractions, as the length of the muscle does not change during these types of contractions.

Dynamic contractions are those that generate force to move an object. The muscle changes in length during these contractions. Contractions that produce a lengthening of the muscle are termed eccentric, whereas those involving muscle shortening are termed concentric. Additionally, if the movement involves a fixed amount of resistance, it is called an isotonic contraction, and if movement takes place at a fixed speed, it is termed an isokinetic contraction. Chapter 20 of *ACSM's Resource Manual for Guidelines for Exercise Testing and Prescription* contains a more thorough overview of factors related to muscular contractions.

FAMILIARIZATION

Some assessment procedures for muscular fitness may require tasks that are uncommon and infrequently performed by the client. Like many other activities, a person's performance can be improved through learning and practicing a technique. This is often called a learning effect. Thus, many muscular fitness assessments will actually require a period of time to teach and familiarize the client with the procedures. Failure to account for this familiarization will affect the accuracy of the assessment results.

Another factor related to client performance is a warm-up prior to participation in the muscular fitness assessments. Beyond the physiologic factors of increasing blood circulation to the muscles and increasing the temperature of the muscles, a warm-up allows a familiarization refresher immediately prior to the assessment.

METHOD OF LOADING

The two major methods employed when applying resistance to the muscle for dynamic contractions are free weights and resistance exercise machines. Each has advantages and disadvantages, both for assessment and training. Among the advantages for free weights are uniformity (i.e., a 25-pound weight plate is the same at every facility), the wide range of movement patterns that can be performed, and their similarity to everyday

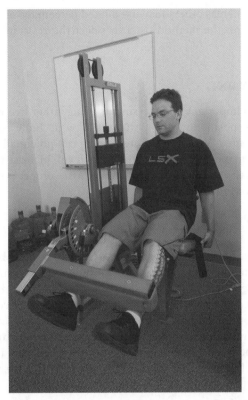

FIGURE 5.1. An example of a resistance exercise unit that utilizes a weight stack for loading.

activities (e.g., lifting and putting a 25-pound box on an overhead shelf). The disadvantages to free weights for assessment purposes are potential difficulty in isolating a muscle group and safety issues related to dropping the weights.

Resistance exercise machines with supported weights, as shown in Figure 5.1, generally can overcome the disadvantages of free weights by limiting a contraction to a specific pattern to better isolate a muscle group and by eliminating the risk to the client from a dropped weight. However, their disadvantages are that movement patterns are limited to one per machine, these isolated patterns are not necessarily typical of everyday activities, and there can be significant variability in the designated amount of weight between different brands of machines (e.g., some machines only use a 1, 2, 3, 4. . . system to designate a difference in load). Also, many machines have some type of mechanism that varies the resistance applied throughout the range of motion of the contraction. Different manufacturers have different mechanisms of varying the resistance. Obviously, this creates difficulties in comparing results from assessments performed on different resistance exercise machines. Also, the ability to track an individual over the course of many years can be affected if the machines used by a facility are upgraded with new models. This issue can be addressed by performing a comparison check on the old versus the new equipment to determine what differences, if any, may exist. If differences are found, a correction factor can be developed, allowing for a more accurate comparison.

In muscular endurance testing, some of the assessments use an individual's body weight as the source of the resistance. Additionally, some tests employ a fixed amount of absolute weight, whereas others may use a fixed percentage of a person's maximum capacity. Depending on the method used to select the resistance, the outcome will vary.

PROPER POSITIONING

Proper positioning is important for assessments using either free weights or machines. Standardization of the positioning is important to allow accurate assessment of the muscle group being measured. Variations in positioning can potentially allow other muscle groups to contribute to movement of the load, which will increase the amount of weight recorded for the assessment, making it inaccurate. Also, proper positioning may be important for the safety of the client.

SPECIFICITY

Typically the principle of specificity is applied to exercise training by tailoring the training exercises to mimic the activity for which an individual is training. Specificity also has relevance for assessment by considering some of the factors mentioned above. The strength or endurance of a muscle will be specific to the type of contraction, the exact movement pattern (or the joint angle for a static measure), the speed of the movement, and the amount of resistance for the endurance measures. Because these specificity characteristics vary between different muscular fitness assessment procedures, interpretation of test results becomes challenging. One key for HRPF assessment of muscular fitness is standardization within the measurement procedure.

MUSCULAR FITNESS CONTINUUM

Muscular fitness is the term used to describe overall ability on the continuum of muscular performance where strength and endurance represent the polar ends of this continuum. From an assessment perspective, strength is the measurement of the maximal force capability of the muscle and endurance is the measurement of the ability to continue performing a contraction at a submaximal level.

STRENGTH ASSESSMENTS

The assessment of muscular strength will be specific to the muscle group and the other unique assessment factors reviewed above. Thus, there is no one single measure of muscular strength for an individual. The best-case scenario for HRPF assessment of muscular strength would be to utilize an assessment of a group of different muscles in some sort of composite score to capture a concept of overall strength of an individual. However, even this approach would be limited in the case of a person with excellent strength levels in some muscles and poor strength levels in other muscles, which would lead to an inaccurate interpretation of average overall muscle strength.

A major decision to be made, which will apply to endurance measurements too, is what method of resistance will be used for the assessments. This decision will be dictated, in part, by the interpretation scale that will be utilized (i.e., if the norms were developed from free weights, then free weights should be used for the assessment).

TABLE 5.1. GRIP-STRENGTH NORMS

AGE (yrs)	15–19		20–29		30–39	
GENDER	M	F	M	F	M	F
Above average	103–112	64–70	113–123	65–70	113–122	66–72
Average	95–102	59–63	106–112	61–64	105–112	61–65
Below average	84–94	54–58	97–105	55–60	97–104	56–60
Poor	≤83	≤53	≤96	≤54	≤96	≤55

AGE (yrs)	40–49		50–59		60–69	
GENDER	M	F	M	F	M	F
Above average	110–118	65–72	102–109	59–64	98–101	54–59
Average	102–109	59–64	96–101	55–58	86–92	51–53
Below average	94–101	55–58	87–95	51–54	79–85	48–50
Poor	≤93	≤54	≤86	≤50	≤78	≤47

Source: Canadian Physical Activity, Fitness & Lifestyle Approach: CSEP-Health & Fitness Program's Health-Related Appraisal & Counseling Strategy, 3rd ed. 2003, 7–47 and 7–48 pp. Reprinted with permission from the Canadian Society for Exercise Physiology.

STATIC

Historically, static measures, particularly of grip strength, have been utilized for many years with origins in physical education classes. However, a variety of different static measures can be performed using either dynamometers or tensiometers. These tests were popular and widely used in physical education programs owing to their low cost and durability.

Dynamometers

The most commonly performed static strength test is the measurement of grip strength using a handgrip dynamometer. Grip-strength norms are given in Table 5.1, and the procedures for the grip-strength test are described in Box 5.1 and illustrated in Figure 5.2.

Another test that has recently been used in fitness settings is the assessment of static back and leg strength. An example of the type of dynamometer used for this assessment is shown in Figure 5.3.

Tensiometers

Another popular form of static strength assessment employs a cable tensiometer. These units can be adjusted to test multiple joint angles through a range of motion for a particular muscular contraction. They can be mounted to walls or tables and can be set up to mimic a variety of common activities. These were more popular in sports-related physical fitness and therefore will not be discussed in more detail in this manual.

DYNAMIC

As reviewed above, dynamic muscular contractions can be performed with either concentric or eccentric movements and with different methods of loading the resistance.

| BOX 5.1 | Procedures for the Static Handgrip Strength Test |

1. Have the client stand for the test. Usually this test is performed with each hand. The norms provided use a combined score for the right and left hands. The test can also be performed with only the dominant hand.
2. Adjust the grip bar so that the second joint of the fingers will be bent to grip the handle of the dynamometer.
3. Have the client hold the handgrip dynamometer parallel to the side of the body. The elbow should be flexed at 90 degrees. Make sure that the dynamometer is set to zero.
4. The client should then squeeze the handgrip dynamometer as hard as possible without holding the breath (to avoid the Valsalva maneuver). It is optional if the client wishes to extend the elbow; however, other body movement should be avoided.
5. Record the grip strength in kilograms. Repeat this procedure using the opposite hand.
6. Repeat the test two more times with each hand. Take the highest of the three readings for each hand and add these two values (one from each hand) together as the measure of handgrip strength to compare with the norms presented in Table 5.1.

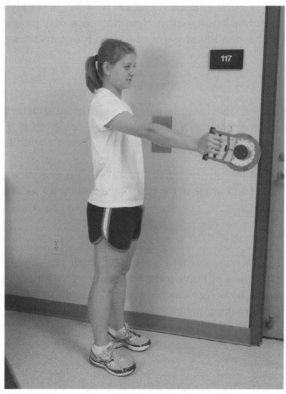

FIGURE 5.2. Measurement of static strength with a handgrip dynamometer.

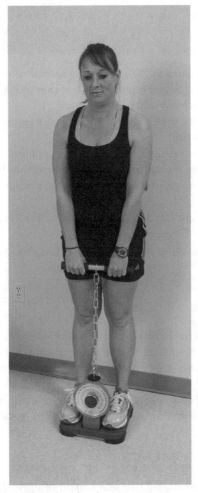

FIGURE 5.3. Measurement of back strength with a dynamometer.

Repetition Maximum

The term used to describe the maximal amount of weight that can be lifted with one contraction is called the repetition maximum (RM). The 1-RM is typically considered the gold standard measure of muscular strength (2). Some fitness professionals have developed strength assessment protocols using multiple repetitions (e.g., 3-RM, 5-RM, 10-RM); however, there are no clear standards or norms available for these evaluations. Likewise, there are some equations to predict a 1-RM value from these multiple-RM tests (4).

The 1-RM test can be performed with any muscle group and can be tested using either free weights or machines. The procedures for performing a 1-RM assessment are provided in Box 5.2. Among the more common exercises used for HRPF assessment are the bench press and the leg press. Tables 5.2 and 5.3 provide normative reference data for these two tests.

BOX 5.2	**Procedures for a One-repetition Maximum (1-RM) Assessment (7)**

1. The subject should warm up by completing several submaximal repetitions.
2. Determine the 1-RM (or any multiple-RM) within four trials with rest periods of 3 to 5 minutes between trials.
3. Select an initial weight that is within the subject's perceived capacity (~50%–70% of capacity).
4. Progressively increase resistance by 2.5–20 kg until the subject cannot complete the selected repetition(s); all repetitions should be performed at the same speed of movement and range of motion to ensure consistency between trials.
5. Record the final weight lifted successfully as the absolute 1-RM or multiple-RM.

American College of Sports Medicine. *ACSM's Guidelines for Exercise Testing and Prescription,* 8th ed. Philadelphia (PA): Wolters Kluwer Health Ltd: 2009, 90 p.

Isokinetic

Isokinetic assessments of muscular fitness require specialized and expensive equipment. The assessments can include a wide range of data that prove highly reliable and accurate. These tests are commonly performed in both athletic and physical therapy rehabilitative programs. However, because of the expense of the equipment and the relatively long time period required to complete an assessment of one muscle group, this type of assessment is not commonly performed in HRPF assessment programs.

ENDURANCE ASSESSMENTS

Like muscular strength assessment, the assessment of muscular endurance will be specific to the muscle group and the other unique assessment factors reviewed above. Endurance assessments can be conducted by performing a fixed amount of contractions in a defined time period, by performing a maximal number of contractions of a set resistance, or by holding a static contraction for a period of time.

DYNAMIC

Dynamic tests of muscular endurance can be performed with free weights or resistance exercise machines. Additionally, these tests can be performed using calisthenic-type exercises, which were popular in physical education classes. This section will cover some of the more common endurance tests that have been utilized, which have normative values for interpretation. However, fitness professionals often create their own tests and can use these as serial assessments over time with a client.

YMCA Submaximal Bench Press Test

This test provides a standardized method to quantify muscular endurance using the bench press exercise. The procedures for this test are provided in Box 5.3 and interpretative norms are located in Table 5.4. Other variations of this test that are sometimes

TABLE 5.2. UPPER BODY STRENGTH[a] NORMS

MALES

Bench Press Weight Ratio = $\dfrac{\text{weight pushed in lbs}}{\text{body weight in lbs}}$

%	<20	20–29	30–39	40–49	50–59	60+	
99	>1.76	>1.63	>1.35	>1.20	>1.05	>.94	
95	1.76	1.63	1.35	1.20	1.05	.94	S
90	1.46	1.48	1.24	1.10	.97	.89	
85	1.38	1.37	1.17	1.04	.93	.84	
80	1.34	1.32	1.12	1.00	.90	.82	E
75	1.29	1.26	1.08	.96	.87	.79	
70	1.24	1.22	1.04	.93	.84	.77	
65	1.23	1.18	1.01	.90	.81	.74	
60	1.19	1.14	.98	.88	.79	.72	G
55	1.16	1.10	.96	.86	.77	.70	
50	1.13	1.06	.93	.84	.75	.68	
45	1.10	1.03	.90	.82	.73	.67	
40	1.06	.99	.88	.80	.71	.66	F
35	1.01	.96	.86	.78	.70	.65	
30	.96	.93	.83	.76	.68	.63	
25	.93	.90	.81	.74	.66	.60	
20	.89	.88	.78	.72	.63	.57	P
15	.86	.84	.75	.69	.60	.56	
10	.81	.80	.71	.65	.57	.53	
5	.76	.72	.65	.59	.53	.49	
1	<.76	<.72	<.65	<.59	<.53	<.49	VP
n	60	425	1,909	2,090	1,279	343	

Total n = 6,106

FEMALES

%	<20	20–29	30–39	40–49	50–59	60+	
99	>.88	>1.01	>.82	>.77	>.68	>.72	
95	.88	1.01	.82	.77	.68	.72	S
90	.83	.90	.76	.71	.61	.64	
85	.81	.83	.72	.66	.57	.59	
80	.77	.80	.70	.62	.55	.54	E
75	.76	.77	.65	.60	.53	.53	
70	.74	.74	.63	.57	.52	.51	
65	.70	.72	.62	.55	.50	.48	
60	.65	.70	.60	.54	.48	.47	G
55	.64	.68	.58	.53	.47	.46	
50	.63	.65	.57	.52	.46	.45	
45	.60	.63	.55	.51	.45	.44	
40	.58	.59	.53	.50	.44	.43	F

(continue)

TABLE 5.2. UPPER BODY STRENGTH[a] NORMS (Continued)

			FEMALES				
35	.57	.58	.52	.48	.43	.41	
30	.56	.56	.51	.47	.42	.40	
25	.55	.53	.49	.45	.41	.39	
20	.53	.51	.47	.43	.39	.38	P
15	.52	.50	.45	.42	.38	.36	
10	.50	.48	.42	.38	.37	.33	
5	.41	.44	.39	.35	.31	.26	
1	<.41	<.44	<.39	<.35	<.31	<.26	VP
n	20	191	379	333	189	42	
Total n = 1,154							

[a]One repetition maximum bench press, with bench press weight ratio = weight pushed in pounds/body weight in pounds.

The Cooper Institute for Aerobics Research. *Physical Fitness Assessments and Norms for Adults and Law Enforcement,* 2002. Available online at http://www.cooperinstitute.org, with permission.

American College of Sports Medicine. *ACSM's Guidelines for Exercise Testing and Prescription,* 8th ed. Philadelphia (PA): Wolters Kluwer Health Ltd: 2009, 91–92 p.

used assess the number of repetitions a person can perform at a certain percentage of his or her 1-RM.

Field Tests

Field tests are particularly useful when testing a large number of people at one time, which is one reason they became popular in physical education classes. Additionally, these tests

TABLE 5.3. LEG STRENGTH NORMS[a]

	AGE				
PERCENTILE	20–29	30–39	40–49	50–59	60+
Men					
90	2.27	2.07	1.92	1.80	1.73
80	2.13	1.93	1.82	1.71	1.62
70	2.05	1.85	1.74	1.64	1.56
60	1.97	1.77	1.68	1.58	1.49
50	1.91	1.71	1.62	1.52	1.43
40	1.83	1.65	1.57	1.46	1.38
30	1.74	1.59	1.51	1.39	1.30
20	1.63	1.52	1.44	1.32	1.25
10	1.51	1.43	1.35	1.22	1.16
Women					
90	1.82	1.61	1.48	1.37	1.32
80	1.68	1.47	1.37	1.25	1.18
70	1.58	1.39	1.29	1.17	1.13
60	1.50	1.33	1.23	1.10	1.04
50	1.44	1.27	1.18	1.05	0.99
40	1.37	1.21	1.13	0.99	0.93
30	1.27	1.15	1.08	0.95	0.88
20	1.22	1.09	1.02	0.88	0.85
10	1.14	1.00	0.94	0.78	0.72

[a]One repetition maximum leg press with leg press weight ratio = weight pushed/body weight.

The Cooper Institute for Aerobics Research. *Physical Fitness Assessments and Norms for Adults and Law Enforcement,* 2002. Available online at http://www.cooperinstitute.org, with permission.

American College of Sports Medicine. *ACSM's Guidelines for Exercise Testing and Prescription,* 8th ed. Philadelphia (PA): Wolters Kluwer Health Ltd: 2009, 92 p.

BOX 5.3	Procedures for the YMCA Submaximal Bench Press Test (5)

The test requires a 35-pound bar for women and a bar with weights totaling 80 pounds for men.

1. Position the client on the bench with both feet on the floor.
2. A spotter should hand the barbell to the client (hands shoulder width apart) and be available throughout the test to grasp the barbell when necessary. The test is started in the down position with the bar touching the chest.
3. Set a metronome to 60 beats per minute and have the client perform a contraction by lifting the bar to full extension with one beat and then lowering the bar to touch the chest with the next beat. The lifting cadence will produce 30 repetitions per minute.
4. The test continues until the client cannot complete a repetition on schedule with the cadence while using correct form. (Note: For highly fit subjects, an upper limit may need to be established.)

Results are compared with the norms presented in Table 5.4.

do not require any equipment and thus can be performed in many different locations, including at home. The two most common field tests are the push-up test and the curl-up test. There are different procedural options (see Fig. 5.4 for an example) available for the test, some of which count the number of repetitions completed in a fixed period of time. It is important to follow the procedures used to establish the normative values that will be used for interpretation. The procedures for the push-up test are provided in Box 5.4 and

TABLE 5.4. YMCA BENCH PRESS TEST—TOTAL LIFTS

CATEGORY	AGE											
	18–25		26–35		36–45		46–55		56–65		>65	
SEX	M	F	M	F	M	F	M	F	M	F	M	F
Excellent	64	66	61	62	55	57	47	50	41	42	36	30
	44	42	41	40	36	33	28	29	24	24	20	18
Good	41	38	37	34	32	30	25	24	21	21	16	16
	34	30	30	29	26	26	21	20	17	17	12	12
Above average	33	28	29	28	25	24	20	18	14	14	10	10
	29	25	26	24	22	21	16	14	12	12	9	8
Average	28	22	24	22	21	20	14	13	11	10	8	7
	24	20	21	18	18	16	12	10	9	8	7	5
Below average	22	18	20	17	17	14	11	9	8	6	6	4
	20	16	17	14	14	12	9	7	5	5	4	3
Poor	17	13	16	13	12	10	8	6	4	4	3	2
	13	9	12	9	9	6	5	2	2	2	2	0
Very poor	<10	6	9	6	6	4	2	1	1	1	1	0

M, male. F, female.

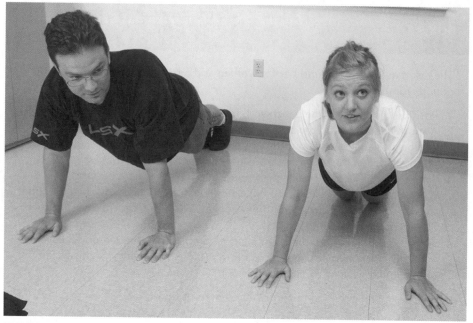

FIGURE 5.4. Different starting positions for men and women for the push-up test.

BOX 5.4	**Push-up Test Procedures for Measurement of Muscular Endurance**

PUSH-UP

1. The push-up test is administered with male subjects starting in the standard "down" position (hands pointing forward and under the shoulder, back straight, head up, using the toes as the pivotal point) and female subjects in the modified "knee push-up" position (legs together, lower leg in contact with mat with ankles plantar-flexed, back straight, hands shoulder width apart, head up, using the knees as the pivotal point).
2. The subject must raise the body by straightening the elbows and return to the "down" position, until the chin touches the mat. The stomach should not touch the mat.
3. For both men and women, the subject's back must be straight at all times and the subject must push up to a straight arm position.
4. The maximal number of push-ups performed consecutively without rest is counted as the score.
5. The test is stopped when the client strains forcibly or is unable to maintain the appropriate technique within two repetitions.

Source: Canadian Physical Activity, Fitness & Lifestyle Approach: CSEP-Health & Fitness Program's Health-Related Appraisal & Counseling Strategy, 3rd ed. 2003, 7–40 p. Reprinted with permission from the Canadian Society for Exercise Physiology.

BOX 5.5	Curl-up (Crunch) Test Procedures for Measurement of Muscular Endurance

CURL-UP (CRUNCH)

1. The individual assumes a supine position on a mat with the knees at 90 degrees. The arms are at the side, palms facing down with the middle fingers touching a piece of masking tape. A second piece of masking tape is placed 10 cm apart.[a] Shoes remain on during the test.
2. A metronome is set to 50 beats · min^{-1} and the individual does slow, controlled curl-ups to lift the shoulder blades off the mat (trunk makes a 30-degree angle with the mat) in time with the metronome at a rate of 25 per minute. The test is done for 1 minute. The low back should be flattened before curling up.
3. Individual performs as many curl-ups as possible without pausing, to a maximum of 25.[b]

[a]Alternatives include (a) having the hands held across the chest, with the head activating a counter when the trunk reaches a 30-degree position (3) and placing the hands on the thighs and curling up until the hands reach the knee caps (5). Elevation of the trunk to 30 degrees is the important aspect of the movement.

[b]An alternative includes doing as many curl-ups as possible in 1 minute.

Source: Canadian Physical Activity, Fitness & Lifestyle Approach: CSEP-Health & Fitness Program's Health-Related Appraisal & Counseling Strategy, 3rd ed. 2003, 7–47 and 7–48 pp. Reprinted with permission from the Canadian Society for Exercise Physiology.

those for the curl-up test are displayed in Box 5.5. Normative data for interpretation of test results are found in Tables 5.5 and 5.6.

STATIC

Another option for muscular endurance assessment is the use of timed tests of holding a submaximal contraction. Some versions of these tests can be created by fitness

TABLE 5.5. FITNESS CATEGORIES FOR PUSH-UP

CATEGORY	AGE									
	20–29		30–39		40–49		50–59		60–69	
SEX	M	F	M	F	M	F	M	F	M	F
Excellent	36	30	30	27	25	24	21	21	18	17
Very good	35	29	29	26	24	23	20	20	17	16
	29	21	22	20	17	15	13	11	11	12
Good	28	20	21	19	16	14	12	10	10	11
	22	15	17	13	13	11	10	7	8	5
Fair	21	14	16	12	12	10	9	6	7	4
	17	10	12	8	10	5	7	2	5	2
Needs improvement	16	9	11	7	9	4	6	1	4	1

Source: Canadian Physical Activity, Fitness & Lifestyle Approach: CSEP-Health & Fitness Program's Health-Related Appraisal & Counseling Strategy, 3rd ed. 2003, 7–47 and 7–48 pp. Reprinted with permission from the Canadian Society for Exercise Physiology.

TABLE 5.6. FITNESS CATEGORIES FOR PARTIAL CURL-UP

| CATEGORY | AGE | | | | | | | | | |
| | 20–29 | | 30–39 | | 40–49 | | 50–59 | | 60–69 | |
SEX	M	F	M	F	M	F	M	F	M	F
Excellent	25	25	25	25	25	25	25	25	25	25
Very good	24	24	24	24	24	24	24	24	24	24
	21	18	18	19	18	19	17	19	16	17
Good	20	17	17	18	17	18	16	18	15	16
	16	14	15	10	13	11	11	10	11	8
Fair	15	13	14	9	12	10	10	9	10	7
	11	5	11	6	6	4	8	6	6	3
Needs improvement	10	4	10	5	5	3	7	5	5	2

Source: Canadian Physical Activity, Fitness & Lifestyle Approach: CSEP-Health & Fitness Program's Health-Related Appraisal & Counseling Strategy, 3e. 2003, 7–47 and 7–48 pp. Reprinted with permission from the Canadian Society for Exercise Physiology.

professionals and used in serial assessments over time with a client. One standardized version of a static muscular endurance test is the timed flexed arm hang. The procedures for this test are provided in Box 5.6, although norms for this test are not well established.

INTERPRETATION ISSUES

There are several issues that complicate the interpretation of results of muscular fitness assessments. The unique assessment issues address several confounding factors including different types of contractions for each muscle, the possibility of a learning curve, improper positioning to allow accessory muscles to contribute to the force, and differences between various methods of loading the resistance. Owing to these multiple factors, a standardized assessment of muscular strength and/or muscular endurance has not been developed.

This chapter provides a variety of different assessment procedures that have been used for many years and for which some normative data exist. These normative data allow for interpretation of the muscular strength and muscular endurance of certain muscles. When using these tables of normative data, it is critical to follow the standardized

---

BOX 5.6	Procedures for the Flexed-arm Hang Test

1. The client stands on a movable box positioned beneath the bar and grasps the bar with an overhand grip (palms facing away) in a position in which the chin is above the bar, elbows are flexed, and the chest is next to the bar.
2. With the client grasping the bar the box is slid away and a stopwatch is started.
3. The position is held as long as possible.
4. The time is stopped when the chin touches the bar and dips below the bar or the head tilts back to keep the chin above the bar.

procedures, which includes using the same equipment as was used by the population on whom the norms were developed. This may be difficult when resistance exercise machines are used to develop the normative chart. A case in point is found with Table 5.3, which provides data for the leg press. These data were developed using the cohort from the Cooper Clinic, which is a large data set from the population tested at this popular center in Dallas, Texas. The data were originally derived from assessments performed using the Universal DSR multistation resistance machines, which were widely available for a period of time. However, as the manufacturers of resistance exercise machines developed newer equipment, these Universal machines were phased out and now are no longer available for purchase. This leads to a dilemma in how to compare and thus assess clients tested with free weights or other brands of resistance exercise machines. Although the American College of Sports Medicine (ACSM) continues to use this as the primary interpretation chart for this test with the presumption that the weight-press ratio will be similar using other equipment, caution must be exercised as this has not been objectively validated.

a   Another issue that is debated is whether to use absolute amounts of weight lifted or to make the amount of weight lifted a proportion of the client's body weight. The norms developed for the bench press and leg press use the ratio method for interpreting the results.

Owing to the limitations in having acceptable norms for interpretation, many fitness professionals forego the process of trying to provide a baseline test interpretation. Instead, the baseline data is only used as a reference point for an individual client, for which future assessments will be compared. Obviously, this does not allow an individual to know how he or she compares to others in the same age group or to a criterion reference standard. Hopefully, with the national recommendations to incorporate resistance exercise into all adults' exercise programs, the development of a national testing battery with interpretation standards for muscular fitness will follow.

SUMMARY

There are several unique factors that do not allow for one single measurement to be made to determine muscular strength or to determine muscular endurance. There are, however, several established tests for the assessment of muscular fitness. The importance of this component of HRPF is growing with the increased emphasis on muscular fitness throughout the lifespan.

> > > **LABORATORY ACTIVITIES**

ASSESSMENT OF MUSCULAR STRENGTH

Data Collection
Work in groups of two or three. If you're working in a group of three, one person will be the subject, another the technician, and another the recorder. Rotate responsibilities until each person has had a chance to serve in each role. Collect the following data on one other member in your group. Record your values on your data sheet.

Hand-grip dynamometer (kg):

	Right	Left	
Trial 1:	_____	_____	
Trial 2:	_____	_____	
Trial 3:	_____	_____	
Best Score:	_____	_____	Sum: _____
Rating (Table 5.1):	_____	_____	

Upper body strength:

1-RM (lbs): _____
Body weight (lbs): _____
Bench press/weight ratio: _____
Percentile ranking (Table 5.2): _____

Lower body strength:

1-RM (lbs): _____
Leg press/weight ratio: _____
Percentile ranking (Table 5.3): _____

Laboratory Report
A. Describe your overall muscular strength based on these three measurements. Explain any limitations that apply to making this interpretation of overall muscular strength.
B. Locate a different set of norms for these three tests. How do the interpretations differ between the norms from the tables in this manual and the ones you found? Be sure to include the reference for the other set of norms.

MUSCULAR ENDURANCE ASSESSMENT

Data Collection
Work in groups of two or three. If you're working in a group of three, one person will be the subject, another the technician, and another the recorder. Rotate responsibilities until each person has had a chance to serve in each role. Collect the following data on one other member in your group. Record your values on your data sheet.

Curl-ups:

Number of curl-ups (max. = 25): _____
Percentile ranking (Table 5.6): _____

Push-ups:

Number of push-ups: _____

Percentile ranking (Table 5.5): _____

YMCA bench press test:

Number of repetitions: _____

Percentile ranking (Table 5.4): _____

Laboratory Report

A. Describe your overall muscular endurance based on these three measurements. Explain any limitations that apply to making this interpretation of overall muscular endurance.

B. Locate a different set of norms for these three tests. How do the interpretations differ between the norms from the tables in this manual and the ones you found? Be sure to include the reference for the other set of norms.

> > > **CASE STUDY**

Bob, who weighs 175 pounds, and Tom, who weighs 225 pounds, have become weight-lifting partners and have been training together for the past 6 months. Bob is 33 years old and Tom is 28 years old. They both completed strength assessments of 1-RM for the bench press and were able to lift 200 pounds on the bench press, whereas Tom lifted 400 pounds on the leg press compared to Bob's 350-pound leg-press performance. Discuss how you would compare and interpret Bob and Tom's muscular strength.

REFERENCES

1. American College of Sports Medicine. Position stand on progression models in resistance training for healthy adults. *Med Sci Sports Exerc.* 2002;34(2):364–80.
2. Fernandez R. One repetition maximum clarified. *J Orthop Sports Phys Ther.* 2001;31:264.
3. Diener MH, Golding LA, Diener D. Validity and reliability of a one-minute half sit-up test of abdominal muscle strength and endurance. *Sports Med Training Rehab.* 1995;6:5–119.
4. Dohoney P, Chromiak JA, Lemire D, et al. Prediction of one repetition maximum (1-RM) strength from a 4-6 RM and 7-10 RM submaximal strength test in healthy young adult males. *J Exerc Physiol Online.* 2002;5:54–9.
5. Faulkner RA, Sprigings EJ, McQuarrie A, et al. A partial curl-up protocol for adults based on an analysis of two procedures. *Can J Sports Sci.* 1989;14:135–41.
6. Golding LA, editor. YMCA Fitness Testing and Assessment Manual. Champaign (IL): *Human Kinetics*; 1989; 167–168 pp.
7. Logan P, Fornasiero D. Abernathy P. Protocols for the assessment of isoinertial strength. In: Fore CJ, ed. Physiological tests for elite athletes. Champaign (IL): *Human Kinetics*; 2000, 200–221 pp.

Flexibility

FLEXIBILITY AS A COMPONENT OF HEALTH-RELATED PHYSICAL FITNESS

Flexibility assessment is an important component of health-related physical fitness (HRPF), as inadequate flexibility decreases performance activities of daily living. Additionally, poor lower back and hip flexibility may contribute to the development of lower back pain, which is one of the more costly medical issues faced by many adults.

Determining flexibility of specific joints is an important part of an HRPF assessment. As with other HRPF measures, flexibility measures are useful as baseline measures to allow comparison of changes following a training program or serially over time as one ages. These baseline and periodic assessments can also identify joints with below desirable levels of flexibility, which can then be targeted for improvement in exercise training programs. Additionally, these assessments may identify strength imbalances in the muscles functioning about the joint. When assessing joint range of motion (ROM), bilateral comparison can identify differences in ROM between the left and right structures being evaluated. ROM deviations may lead to muscle imbalances and cause adjacent joint and muscle structures to overcompensate within the kinetic chain of movement, resulting in dysfunction within the related joint structures and the potential to develop injuries, trauma, and movement pattern complications.

UNIQUE ASSESSMENT PRINCIPLES

Flexibility is the functional capacity of the joints to move through a full ROM. The gold standard for determining flexibility is the laboratory assessment of the ROM of a specific joint. As was the case for muscular fitness, there are literally hundreds of joints in the human body, each of which can have a different level of flexibility. Indeed, entire manuals have been devoted to assessment of ROM of the human body joints (3,4). Two requirements of any flexibility assessment are that it be specific to a joint and that an adequate warm-up is provided for the client.

SPECIFICITY

Flexibility will vary depending on which muscle and joint are being evaluated (i.e., it is joint specific), which essentially rules out the possibility of a single test that can truly characterize one's flexibility. Additionally, each joint has a set ROM that is unique to the function of the specific joint.

WARM-UP

An adequate warm-up is essential prior to assessing flexibility. The warm-up should begin with some whole body aerobic exercise such as walking or cycling as shown in Figure 6.1, ideally involving both arms and legs, to increase blood flow and temperature. The aerobic warm-up should then be followed by some passive stretching and ROM exercises of the joints to be assessed.

METHODS OF MEASUREMENT

Many different methods are used for assessing flexibility. These range from fairly simple visual methods, to measuring the change in distance, to using specially designed devices

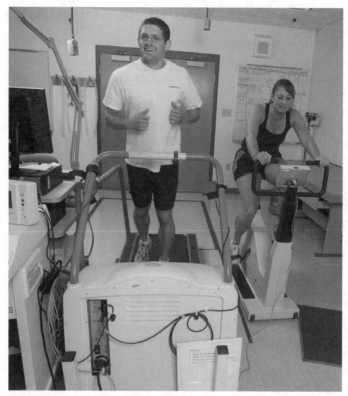

FIGURE 6.1. A flexibility assessment should be preceded by a warm-up period that could include walking or cycling.

to assess ROM, including new technology that uses digital video cameras and software. The most widely used device for determining ROM is a goniometer, with some such instruments using an electronic scale (electrogoniometers). The goniometer measurement of joint movement in degrees is considered the gold standard measure for flexibility assessment. Other devices for flexibility assessment include the Leighton flexometer and inclinometers.

This manual will focus on the assessment of some of the major joints in the body that are used to perform physical activities and exercise for health-related reasons. Assessments made both with measures of distance and with a goniometer will be reviewed.

DISTANCE TESTS FOR ASSESSMENT OF FLEXIBILITY

SIT-AND-REACH TEST

Probably the most widely used flexibility test in physical fitness programs is the sit-and-reach test. This test became popular based on the belief that limitations in this bending and reaching movement are associated with low back pain and may predispose one to a low back injury. The procedures for this test are provided in Box 6.1. It should be noted that there are various modifications that have been proposed for the sit-and-reach test; however, norms for all these variations are not well established.

BOX 6.1   Procedures for Sit and Reach Test

Pretest: Participant should perform a short warm-up before this test and include some stretches (e.g., modified hurdler's stretch). It is also recommended that the participant refrain from fast, jerky movements, which may increase the possibility of an injury. The participant's shoes should be removed.

1. For the Canadian Trunk Forward Flexion test, the client sits without shoes and the soles of the feet flat against the flexometer (sit-and-reach box) at the 26-cm mark. Inner edges of the soles are placed within 2 cm of the measuring scale. For the YMCA sit-and-reach test, a yardstick is placed on the floor and tape is placed across it at a right angle to the 15-inch mark. The participant sits with the yardstick between the legs, with legs extended at right angles to the taped line on the floor. Heels of the feet should touch the edge of the taped line and be about 10 to 12 inches apart. (Note the zero point at the foot/box interface and use the appropriate norms.)
2. The participant should slowly reach forward with both hands as far as possible, holding this position ~2 seconds. Be sure that the participant keeps the hands parallel and does not lead with one hand. Fingertips can be overlapped and should be in contact with the measuring portion or yardstick of the sit-and-reach box.
3. The score is the most distant point (in centimeters or inches) reached with the fingertips. The best of two trials should be recorded. To assist with the best attempt, the participant should exhale and drop the head between the arms when reaching. Testers should ensure that the knees of the participant stay extended; however, the participant's knees should not be pressed down. The participant should breathe normally during the test and should not hold his or her breath at any time. Norms for the Canadian test are presented in Table 6.1. Note that these norms use a sit-and-reach box in which the zero point is set at the 26-cm mark. If you are using a box in which the zero point is set at 23 cm (e.g., Fitnessgram), subtract 3 cm from each value in this table. The norms for the YMCA test are presented in Table 6.2.

Source: YMCA Fitness Testing and Assessment Manual, 4th ed. Chicago (IL): YMCA of the USA, 158–160 pp.

ASSESSMENT OF LUMBAR FLEXION

The lumbar flexion test takes place with the client seated on floor or table with legs extended and pelvis stabilized to prevent anterior/posterior tilting, as depicted in Figure 6.2. Tape is positioned with the zero mark at the spinous process C7 and measurement is taken down to the superior iliac (or level to the posterior superior iliac spine). The client performs lumbar flexion until the first sign of resistance and the increase in distance is recorded. An average range for healthy adults is a 4-inch increase as the spine flexes.

ASSESSMENT OF LUMBAR EXTENSION

The test takes place with the client seated in the same position as was used for lumbar flexion, with the tape positioned in the same starting position, as illustrated in Figure 6.3.

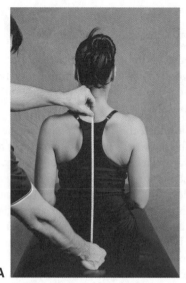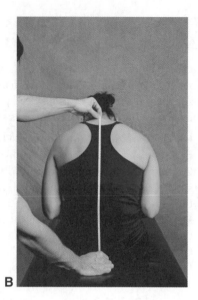

FIGURE 6.2. Assessment of lumbar flexion.

The client performs lumbar extension until the first sign of resistance. An average range for healthy adults is a 2-inch increase as the spine extends.

RANGE OF MOTION DEFINED

Many of the joints of the body can perform several different kinds of movements, in different planes and at different angles, depending on the type of joint structure and its designated function (1). ROM is defined as the amount of available motion, or arc of

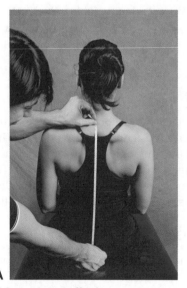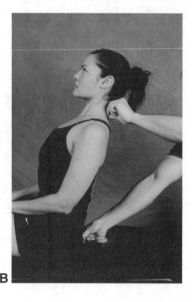

FIGURE 6.3. Assessment of lumbar extension.

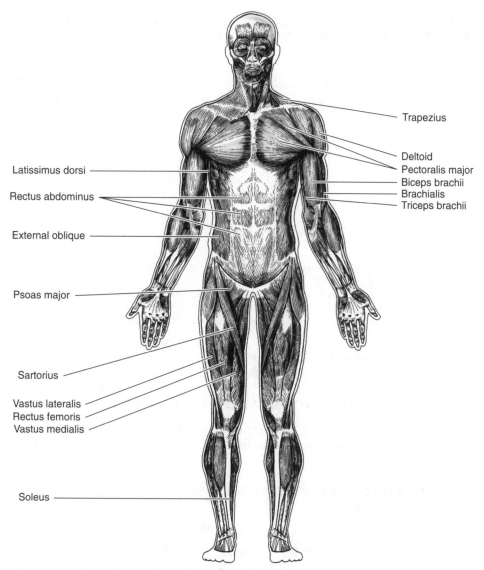

Trapezius

Deltoid
Pectoralis major
Biceps brachii
Brachialis
Triceps brachii

Latissimus dorsi

Rectus abdominus

External oblique

Psoas major

Sartorius

Vastus lateralis
Rectus femoris
Vastus medialis

Soleus

FIGURE 6.4. Anatomic start position.

motion, that occurs at a specific joint (3). All ROM assessments start in the anatomic start position, except motions in rotation. In the anatomic start position, the body is set at 0 degrees of flexion, extension, abduction, and adduction, as displayed in Figure 6.4. ROM can be assessed two ways: active ROM, which is the motion achieved by the client without assistance by an examiner, or passive ROM, which is the motion achieved by an examiner without the assistance from the client. For HRPF assessments, only active ROM exercises are performed. Passive ROM should only be performed by physicians and allied health professionals such as physical therapists, athletic trainers, and kine-siotherapists for specific types of medical evaluations.

The fitness professional should be aware of several key factors known to influence flexibility in adults. Age (flexibility tends to decrease with age), gender (flexibility of specific joints is different), previous injuries to the joint (if structural damage occurred

TABLE 6.1. FITNESS CATEGORIES BY AGE GROUPS FOR TRUNK FORWARD FLEXION USING A SIT-AND-REACH BOX (cm)[a]

CATEGORY	AGE									
	20–29		30–39		40–49		50–59		60–69	
SEX	M	F	M	F	M	F	M	F	M	F
Excellent	40	41	38	41	35	38	35	39	33	35
Very good	39	40	37	40	34	37	34	38	32	34
	34	37	33	36	29	34	28	33	25	31
Good	33	36	32	35	28	33	27	32	24	30
	30	33	28	32	24	30	24	30	20	27
Fair	29	32	27	31	23	29	23	29	19	26
	25	28	23	27	18	25	16	25	15	23
Needs improvement	24	27	22	26	17	24	15	24	14	22

M, male; F, female.

[a]Note: These norms are based on a sit-and-reach box in which the zero point is set at 26 cm. When using a box in which the zero point is set at 23 cm, subtract 3 cm from each value in this table.

Source: Canadian Physical Activity, Fitness & Lifestyle Approach: CSEP-Health & Fitness Program's Health-Related Appraisal & Counseling Strategy, 3rd ed. 2003, 7–47 and 7–48 pp. Reprinted with permission from the Canadian Society for Exercise Physiology.

American College of Sports Medicine. *ACSM's Guidelines for Exercise Testing and Prescription*, 8th ed. Philadelphia (PA): Wolters Kluwer Health Ltd: 2009, 100 p.

or if a surgical procedure was needed), and specific diseases that affect the joint (e.g., arthritis) are all factors that may impact flexibility.

GONIOMETERS—TOOLS TO MEASURE RANGE OF MOTION

The goniometer comes in many different shapes (0–180 degrees or 0–360 degrees), sizes (length of the arms), and materials (metal or plastic). The design of the

TABLE 6.2. PERCENTILES BY AGE GROUPS AND SEX FOR YMCA SIT-AND-REACH TEST (Inches)

PERCENTILE	AGE											
	18–25		26–35		36–45		46–55		56–65		>65	
SEX	M	F	M	F	M	F	M	F	M	F	M	F
90	22	24	21	23	21	22	19	21	17	20	17	20
80	20	22	19	21	19	21	17	20	15	19	15	18
70	19	21	17	20	17	19	15	18	13	17	13	17
60	18	20	17	20	16	18	14	17	13	16	12	17
50	17	19	15	19	15	17	13	16	11	15	10	15
40	15	18	14	17	13	16	11	14	9	14	9	14
30	14	17	13	16	13	15	10	14	9	13	8	13
20	13	16	11	15	11	14	9	12	7	11	7	11
10	11	14	9	13	7	12	6	10	5	9	4	9

M, male; F, female.

The following may be used as descriptors for the percentile rankings: well above average (90), above average (70), average (50), below average (30), and well below average (10).

Reprinted with permission, YMCA Fitness Testing and Assessment Manual, 4th ed. Champaign (IL): Human Kinetics; 2000; 200–211. All rights reserved.

American College of Sports Medicine. *ACSM's Guidelines for Exercise Testing and Prescription*, 8th ed. Philadelphia (PA): Wolters Kluwer Health Ltd: 2009, 101 p.

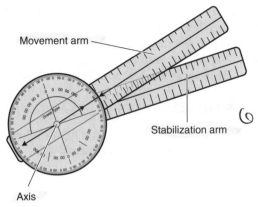

FIGURE 6.5. A goniometer, including the body axis or fulcrum, a stabilization arm, and a movement arm.

goniometer, as seen in Figure 6.5, includes a body, a fulcrum or center point, a stabilization arm, and a movement arm. The body of a goniometer is similar to a protractor and consists of the arc of a circle. Around the circle are degree measurements that will range from either 0–180 degrees or from 0–360 degrees. The fulcrum is centered to the identified anatomic landmark required for a given ROM assessment. The stabilization arm is the body segment of the goniometer that will remain fixed and stable during the test. The stabilization arm establishes the starting position of the measurement. The movement arm is the body segment of the goniometer that will move in relation to the subject's movement during the test. The movement arm is set with the ending position.

RANGE-OF-MOTION ASSESSMENT OVERVIEW

Prior to beginning the assessment, the client should be provided with a demonstration of a sample ROM test on a joint to explain how the assessment works. As each joint's ROM is assessed, the proper starting position, performance of the ROM test, and ending position should all be demonstrated. The following process to position the goniometer occurs before the onset of the assessment:

- Locate the fulcrum at the joint axis or hinge point where the axis of rotation occurs for the two body segments involved.
- Place the stabilization and movement arms so that they are centered along each body segment according to the landmarks for each joint measurement (note that the goniometer arms should be long enough to properly align with the landmarks).

The stationary arm of the goniometer will need to be stabilized while the movement arm moves with the body segment through the ROM. The client should be instructed to move the body segment slowly through the ROM until the body segment cannot move further without compensating the body through shifting or causing discomfort. When there is no further movement, the joint angle is measured and recorded. The use of goniometry can be an accurate measure of a joint's ROM when the following procedures are properly performed (2):

- All anatomic landmarks are identified.
- The joint axis point has been clearly defined.
- The body is stabilized in proper alignment from the start to ending positions.

- The client is instructed to move slowly through the proper ROM, and the goniometer is kept aligned to each body segment.
- Measurements are read and recorded correctly.
- The test administrator is familiar with the normal ROM for each joint structure.
- Careful observations are made as to whether each joint's ROM assessment is pain free.

SPECIFIC RANGE-OF-MOTION TESTS

In all ROM assessments, locations of the goniometer for the following three points need to be clearly specified to ensure accurate measurements:

1. Fulcrum
2. Stabilization arm
3. Movement arm

Additionally, stabilization of surrounding body parts must occur and starting and ending body positions must be defined and measured precisely. Below are specifications for the various ROM assessments of the shoulder and the hip. An average ROM for each assessment is also provided in Table 6.3.

Structure: The Shoulder

Movement: Flexion

Goniometer Position (Fig. 6.6)

1. Fulcrum: Lateral aspect of greater tubercle
2. Stabilization arm: Perpendicular to the floor
3. Movement arm: Aligned with midline of humerus and referenced with the lateral epicondyle

Stabilization: Client is in good posture with a stabilized scapula (retracted) and thoracic and lumbar spine. Stabilize scapula to prevent tilting, rotation, or elevation. *Starting/ending body position:* Client is seated with glenohumeral in 0 degrees of flexion, extension, abduction, or adduction. Head is in neutral position. Palm of hand should face the body. Elbow should be extended completely. Client performs glenohumeral flexion until the first sign of resistance.

TABLE 6.3. AVERAGE RANGE OF MOTION FOR SELECTED FLEXIBILITY ASSESSMENTS

FLEXIBILITY TEST	AVERAGE FOR THIS JOINT'S RANGE OF MOTION
Shoulder flexion	0–180°
Shoulder extension	0–60°
Shoulder internal rotation	0–70°
Shoulder external rotation	0–90°
Hip flexion (testing leg fully extended)	0–90°
Hip flexion (testing knee flexed 90° and hip flexed 90°)	0–120°
Hip extension (testing leg fully extended)	0–30°
Hip abduction	0–45°
Hip adduction	0–30°

ACSM's Health-related Physical Fitness Assessment Manual, 2nd ed. Baltimore (MD): Lippincott, Williams, and Wilkins: 2005, 89–94 pp.

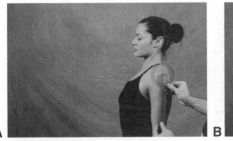
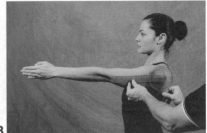

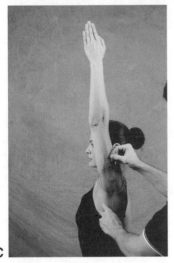

FIGURE 6.6. Shoulder flexion range of motion.

Movement: Extension

Goniometer Position (Fig. 6.7)

1. Fulcrum: Lateral aspect of greater tubercle
2. Stabilization arm: Perpendicular to the floor
3. Movement arm: Aligned with midline of the lateral humerus and referenced with the lateral epicondyle

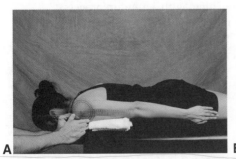
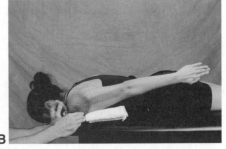

FIGURE 6.7. Shoulder extension range of motion.

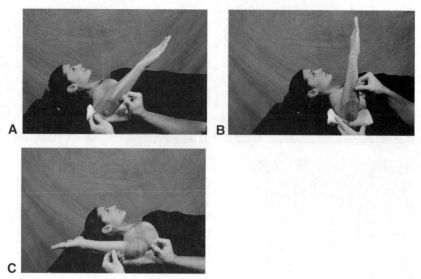

FIGURE 6.8. Shoulder rotation—both internal and external range of motion.

Stabilization: Client is in good posture with a stabilized scapula (retracted) and thoracic and lumbar spine. Stabilize scapula to prevent tilting, rotation, or elevation. Place towel under humerus to stabilize and align with acromion process.
Starting/ending body position: Client is prone on table with glenohumeral in 0 degrees of flexion, extension, abduction, or adduction. Head is in neutral position. Palm of hand should face the body. Elbow should be extended completely. Client performs glenohumeral extension until the first sign of resistance.

Movement: Internal Rotation

Goniometer Position (Fig. 6.8)

1. Fulcrum: Olecranon process of the elbow
2. Stabilization arm: Perpendicular to the floor
3. Movement arm: Aligned with lateral midline of ulna and referenced with the ulnar styloid

Stabilization: Client is in good posture with a stabilized scapula (retracted) and thoracic and lumbar spine. Stabilize scapula to prevent tilting, rotation, or elevation. Place towel under humerus to stabilize and align with acromion process.
Starting/ending body position: Client is supine on table with humerus abducted at 90 degrees and elbow flexed at 90 degrees. Elbow is at 0 degrees of supination and pronation. Client performs glenohumeral internal rotation until the first sign of resistance.

Movement: External Rotation

Goniometer Position

1. Fulcrum: Olecranon process of the elbow
2. Stabilization arm: Perpendicular to the floor

3. Movement arm: Aligned with lateral midline of ulna and referenced with the ulnar styloid

Stabilization: Client is in good posture with a stabilized scapula (retracted) and thoracic and lumbar spine. Stabilize scapula to prevent tilting, rotation, or elevation. Place towel under humerus to stabilize and align with acromion process.

Starting/ending body position: Client is supine on table with humerus abducted at 90 degrees and elbow flexed at 90 degrees. Elbow is at 0 degrees of supination and pronation. Client performs glenohumeral external rotation until the first sign of resistance.

Structure: The Hip

Movement: Flexion (Testing Leg Fully Extended)

Goniometer Position (Fig. 6.9)

1. Fulcrum: Greater trochanter of the lateral thigh
2. Stabilization arm: Lateral midline of the pelvis
3. Movement arm: Lateral midline of the femur, using the lateral epicondyle as a reference

Stabilization: Client is in good posture with a stabilized scapula, thoracic and lumbar spine, and pelvic area. Pelvis should not rise off table. Opposite leg not being assessed should have knee flexed and foot flat on table for added stability and protection for the back.

Starting/ending body position: Client is supine on table with hip in 0 degrees of flexion, extension, abduction, adduction, and rotation. Testing leg has knee fully

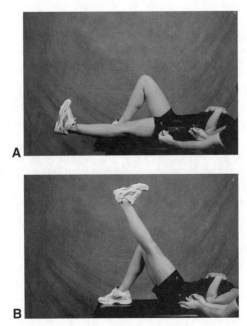

FIGURE 6.9. Hip flexion range of motion (testing leg fully extended).

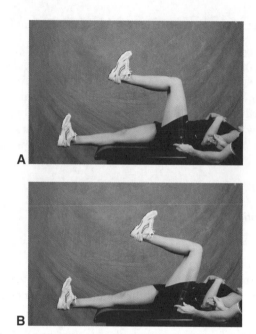

FIGURE 6.10. Hip flexion range of motion (testing knee flexed 90 degrees and hip flexed 90 degrees).

extended. Subject performs hip flexion until the first sign of resistance or until the pelvis rotates or knee breaks extension.

Movement: Flexion (Testing Knee Flexed 90 Degrees and Hip Flexed 90 Degrees)

Goniometer Position (Fig. 6.10)

1. Fulcrum: Greater trochanter of the lateral thigh
2. Stabilization arm: Lateral midline of the pelvis
3. Movement arm: Lateral midline of the femur, using the lateral epicondyle as a reference

Stabilization: Client is in good posture with a stabilized scapula, thoracic and lumbar spine, and pelvic area. Pelvis should not rise off table. Opposite leg not being assessed should have knee extended on table for added stability and protection for the back.

Starting/ending body position: Client is supine on table with knee flexed at 90 degrees and hip flexed at 90 degrees; and hip is in 0 degrees of abduction, adduction, and rotation. Knee is flexed to reduce contraction of hamstrings. Client performs hip flexion until the first sign of resistance or until the pelvis rotates.

Movement: Extension (Testing Leg Fully Extended)

Goniometer Position (Fig. 6.11)

1. Fulcrum: Greater trochanter of the lateral thigh
2. Stabilization arm: Lateral midline of the pelvis

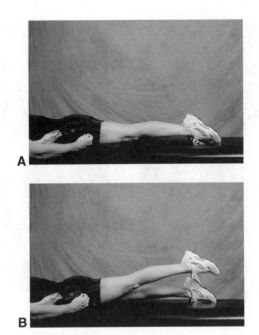

FIGURE 6.11. Hip extension range of motion.

3. Movement arm: Lateral midline of the femur, using the lateral epicondyle as a reference

Stabilization: Client is in good posture with a stabilized scapula, thoracic and lumbar spine, and pelvic area. Pelvis should not rise off table. Opposite leg not being assessed should have leg fully extended on table for added stability.
Starting/ending body position: Client is prone on table with hip in 0 degrees of flexion, extension, abduction, adduction, and rotation. Testing leg has knee fully extended. Client performs hip extension until the first sign of resistance or until the pelvis rotates.

Movement: Abduction

Goniometer Position (Fig. 6.12)

1. Fulcrum: Locate at the anterior superior iliac spine (ASIS)
2. Stabilization arm: Imaginary horizontal line connecting axis point ASIS to the other ASIS
3. Movement arm: Anterior midline of the femur, using the midline of the patella as a reference

Stabilization: Client is in good posture with a stabilized scapula, thoracic and lumbar spine, and pelvic area. Stabilize for lateral trunk flexion on both sides.
Starting/ending body position: Client is supine on table with hip in 0 degrees of flexion, extension, and rotation. Testing leg has knee fully extended. Client performs hip abduction until the first sign of resistance or lateral trunk flexion occurs on either side.

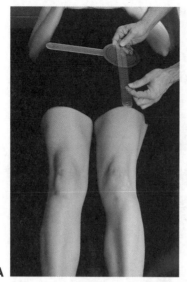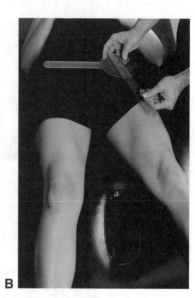

A   **B**

FIGURE 6.12. Hip abduction range of motion.

Movement: Adduction

Goniometer Position

1. Fulcrum: Located at the ASIS
2. Stabilization arm: Imaginary horizontal line connecting axis point ASIS to the other ASIS
3. Movement arm: Anterior midline of the femur, using the midline of the patella as a reference

Stabilization: Client is in good posture with a stabilized scapula, thoracic and lumbar spine, and pelvic area. Opposite leg not being tested should be abducted fully to allow for testing hip to be assessed.

Starting/ending body position: Client is supine on table with hip in 0 degrees of flexion, extension, and rotation. Testing leg has knee fully extended. Client performs hip adduction until the first sign of resistance or lateral trunk flexion or pelvic rotation occurs.

INTERPRETATION

The reference ranges for ROM for the measurements reviewed in this manual are shown in Table 6.3. *ACSM's Guidelines for Exercise Testing and Prescription,* 8th edition (*GETP8*) provides values for other joints in the body.

It is important to recognize that a learning effect is likely with flexibility measurements. Thus, the following statement from *ACSM's Resource Manual for Guidelines for Exercise Testing and Prescription* (p. 344) is of importance:

A recommendation from the American Medical Association (1) suggests that ROM should be measured using three consecutive trials and averaged as the true value. If the average ROM is 50 degrees, three of the measurements must fall within ±5 degrees of the mean. If the average is greater than 50 degrees, three measurements must fall within ±10 degrees of average. Such measures may be taken up to six times until they meet the criteria; otherwise, they are considered invalid.

SUMMARY

Similar to the HRPF assessment of muscular endurance, there is no one single measurement that provides an overall measurement of flexibility. Fortunately, goniometer assessments are quite feasible, which provides a great opportunity to perform these assessments with clients. Fitness professionals are increasingly incorporating flexibility assessments in their evaluation of clients' HRPF.

> > > **LABORATORY ACTIVITIES**

RANGE-OF-MOTION ASSESSMENTS

Data Collection

Work with one other student (he or she measures you, you measure him or her) to perform the ROM assessments listed below. The measure is taken passively as the movement is slowly and gradually performed until maximum range is achieved as evidenced by high mechanical resistance or the discomfort of the subject.

Movement	Right	Left
Hip flexion—testing leg fully extended	_____	_____
Hip flexion—testing knee flexed 90° and hip flexed 90°	_____	_____
Hip extension—testing leg fully extended	_____	_____
Hip adduction	_____	_____
Hip abduction	_____	_____
Shoulder flexion	_____	_____
Shoulder extension	_____	_____
Shoulder internal rotation	_____	_____
Shoulder external rotation	_____	_____

Written Report

Provide an interpretation of your ROM for each measured movement. Highlight any results that were not within the expected average range for each measure. Were there any imbalances between assessments on the right versus the left side of the body? Comment on what problems could arise from poor flexibility test scores from these measurements.

DISTANCE TESTS FOR FLEXIBILITY ASSESSMENT

Data Collection

Work with one other student (he or she measures you, you measure him or her) to perform the distance tests of flexibility assessments listed below. The measure is taken passively as the movement is slowly and gradually performed until maximum range is achieved as evidenced by high mechanical resistance or the discomfort of the subject.

Sit-and-reach Test

Trial 1: _____   Trial 2: _____   Trial 3: _____

Best score: _____

Lumbar flexion:

Trial 1: _____   Trial 2: _____   Trial 3: _____

Best score: _____

Lumbar extension:

Trial 1: _____   Trial 2: _____   Trial 3: _____

Best score: _____

Written Report

Provide an interpretation of your flexibility for each test. Comment on what problems could arise from poor flexibility test scores from these measurements.

> > > **CASE STUDY**

Jill stopped by a booth at a local health fair and had a flexibility assessment. Jill, who is 33 years of age, scored in the well-above-average category for this sit-and-reach test. Jill was given a copy of the report, which stated that her flexibility was "excellent." As her fitness consultant, Jill brings a copy of this report to you. What should you tell Jill about this report and this health-related physical fitness component?

REFERENCES

1. American Medical Association. *Guides to the Evaluation of Permanent Impairment.* 4th ed. Chicago 1993: American Medical Association.
2. Griffin JC. Client-centered musculoskeletal assessments. In: Wilgren S, Mustain E, Grahm M, eds. *Manual of Centered Exercise Prescription.* Champaign (IL) 1998: Human Kinetics.
3. Lea R, Gerhardt J. Current concepts review. Range of motion measurements. *J Bone Joint Surg.* 1995;77(5):784–98.
4. Norkin CC, White DJ. *Measurement of Joint Motion: A Guide to Goniometry.* 2nd ed. Philadelphia 1995: F.A. Davis Co.

Cardiorespiratory Fitness: Estimation from Field and Submaximal Exercise Tests

WHY MEASURE CARDIORESPIRATORY FITNESS?

Cardiorespiratory fitness (CRF) reflects the functional capabilities of the heart, blood vessels, lungs, and skeletal muscles to perform work. CRF is the ability to perform large-muscle, dynamic, moderate- to high-intensity exercise for prolonged periods. There are many different terms that have been used to describe this measure of physical fitness, including:

- Maximal aerobic capacity
- Functional capacity
- Physical work capacity (PWC)
- Cardiovascular endurance, fitness, or capacity
- Cardiorespiratory endurance, fitness, or capacity
- Cardiopulmonary endurance, fitness, or capacity

HEALTH IMPLICATIONS

The assessment of CRF is used for individualizing the exercise prescription, for tracking progress and providing motivation for an individual in an exercise program, and for providing patients with chronic diseases valuable clinical information. As reviewed in Chapter 5 of *ACSM's Guidelines for Exercise Testing and Prescription*, 8th edition (*GETP8*), a low level of CRF has been established as an independent risk factor for all-cause and cardiovascular mortality.

FUNCTIONAL IMPLICATIONS

Another important aspect of CRF is that it directly relates to an individual's functional status, as noted by the use of the term *functional capacity* to describe CRF. This can be demonstrated in part by comparing a 55-year-old man with high CRF fitness (14.2 metabolic equivalents [METs]) to one with low CRF fitness (7.4 METs). The highly fit man can easily perform occupational and recreational activities that require 6–9 METS, such as carrying groceries upstairs, riding a bicycle at 10 mph, shoveling snow, or playing singles tennis (1). The man with low fitness will only be able to be perform these same activities, if at all, with maximal effort.

WHAT IS THE GOLD STANDARD TEST?

The gold standard measure of CRF is the maximal exercise test with collection of expired gases. This test is performed in a laboratory setting, with trained personnel, using specific monitoring equipment. Maximal exercise testing will be covered in Chapter 8. Because this method is the most involved (time and expense) and involves a higher level of risk, it is not always feasible or desired. It should also be noted that maximal exercise testing is also done in clinical settings for diagnosis and prognosis of some chronic diseases. Fortunately, there are many alternative approaches to provide estimates of CRF. These alternative assessment tests for CRF fall into two categories:

1. Field tests: These tests can take place in a variety of nonlaboratory settings (i.e., in the "field") and can typically be administered to a group of people simultaneously. Most commonly, these tests require clients to complete a certain distance as quickly

as possible, or to cover as much distance as possible in a fixed amount of time, or to perform a set amount of work in a fixed amount of time.

2. Submaximal exercise tests: These exercise tests limit the level of effort to submaximal exertion. These tests are typically performed in a laboratory setting by one client at a time.

DECIDING ON WHICH METHOD TO USE

The fitness professional needs to assist the client in determining which test may be the most appropriate for CRF assessment. Because the alternative tests involve the prediction of CRF, the standard error of the estimation (SEE) is part of the decision process. Other factors that may influence the test selection decision are:

- Time required
- Expense
- Personnel needed
- Equipment and facilities needed
- Risk level

PRETEST STANDARDIZATIONS FOR CARDIORESPIRATORY FITNESS ASSESSMENTS

To obtain optimal results, it is important to provide pretest instructions for clients to follow prior to performing a CRF assessment test. Clients should be instructed to wear comfortable exercise-type clothing, avoid tobacco and caffeine 3 hours prior to the test, avoid alcohol 12 hours prior to the test, consume plenty of fluids and avoid strenuous exercise for 24 hours prior to the test, and obtain an adequate amount of sleep the night before the test.

The informed consent process should be completed and performance instructions specific to the test should be reviewed with the client. It is very important that the client understand that he or she is free to terminate the test at any time and is also responsible for informing the test administrator of any and all symptoms that might develop. Also, if used, an explanation of the rating of perceived exertion scale (RPE) is warranted at this time. This scale is provided in Table 4.7 of *ACSM's GETP8*. Verbal directions should be read to the client prior to the test for obtaining the RPE measurement. These directions should be consistent with the recommendations of Borg (2).

FIELD TESTS FOR PREDICTION OF AEROBIC CAPACITY

Many field tests originated from physical education curricula that desired to assess CRF of a large group of students at the same time in a nonlaboratory, or field, setting. Field tests have several advantages. They do not require highly trained personnel to administer them and they are inexpensive, requiring little if any equipment. Generally, these types of tests are considered safe to perform; however, this may be because they are typically used in younger, low-risk populations. It is important to recognize that some of the tests, such as running 1.5 miles as rapidly as possible, will result in a maximal or near-maximal level of exertion. This requirement may be inappropriate for individuals at moderate to high risk for cardiovascular or musculoskeletal complications. The importance of performing the screening procedures reviewed in Chapter 2 on all clients prior to a CRF assessment and following the personnel recommendations (for supervision) are thus warranted.

STEP TESTS

The original Harvard two-step test was first used in medicine to aid in the diagnosis of heart disease (10). Many alternative methods have been developed; however, most are based on the same protocol in which the client performs a fixed amount of work in a set amount of time, followed by the measurement of heart rate response. This manual reviews the McArdle or Queens College step test, which has been commonly used to simultaneously test large groups of students to predict their CRF (9). The procedures for the Queens College step test are provided in Box 7.1. Note, any changes to the procedure, including using a different step height or a different rate of stepping, will invalidate the results.

BOX 7.1   Queens College Step Test Procedures

1. The step test requires that the individual step up and down on a standardized step height of 16.25 in. (41.25 cm) for 3 minutes. (Many gymnasium bleachers have a riser height of 16.25 in.)
2. Men step at a rate (cadence) of 24 per minute, whereas women step at a rate of 22 per minute. This cadence should be closely monitored and set with the use of an electronic metronome. A 24-step-per-minute cadence means that the complete cycle of step up with one leg, step up with the other, step down with the first leg, and finally step down with the last leg is performed 24 times in a minute. Commonly the metronome is set at a cadence of four times the step rate, in this case 96 beats per minute for men, to coordinate each leg's movement with a beat of the metronome. The women's step cadence would be 88 beats per minute. Although it may be possible to test more than one client at a time, the group would need to be of the same gender.
3. At the conclusion of 3 minutes, the client stops and palpates the pulse (typically at the radial site) while standing within the first 5 seconds. A 15-second pulse count is then taken and multiplied by 4 to determine heart rate (HR) in beats per minute (bpm). The recovery HR should occur within the first 30 seconds of immediate recovery from the end of the step test. The subject's $\dot{V}O_{2max}$ is determined from the recovery HR by the following formulas:

$$\text{For men: } \dot{V}O_{2max} (mL \cdot kg^{-1} \cdot min^{-1}) = 111.33 - (0.42 \times HR)$$

$$\text{For Women: } \dot{V}O_{2max} (mL \cdot kg^{-1} \cdot min^{-1}) = 65.81 - (0.1847 \times HR)$$

$$HR = \text{recovery HR (bpm)}$$

For example, if a man finished the test with a recovery HR = 144 bpm (36 beats in 15 s), then:

$$\dot{V}O_{2max} (mL \cdot kg^{-1} \cdot min^{-1}) = 111.33 - (0.42 \times 144) = 50.85 \ mL \cdot kg^{-1} \cdot min^{-1}$$

The Queens College step test is also known as the McArdle step test (9).

FIXED DISTANCE TESTS

There are two common field test protocols that predict CRF by using a walk or run performance of a fixed distance. The performance tests can be classified into two groups: walk/run tests or pure walk tests. In the walk/run test, the subject can walk, run, or use a combination of both to complete the test. In the pure walking tests, subjects are strictly limited to walking the entire test.

The 1-mile walk test is generally indicated for those who have been sedentary or irregularly active or are unable to run because of an injury. The client should be able to walk briskly for 1 mile to be a good candidate for this test.

The 1-mile walk test requires that the subject walk 1 mile as quickly as possible around a measured course. Walking is defined as having one foot in contact with the ground at all times (running involves an airborne phase). The test requires an accurate measure of body weight and a clock to time both the duration of the walk and a 15-second pulse count following the walk. A heart rate monitor is preferred to a pulse count if one is available. Immediately following the 1-mile walk, the time to complete the test and the heart rate (HR) at the end of the test are recorded. If pulse palpation is used, the client counts the recovery pulse for 15 seconds and multiplies by 4 to determine a 1-minute recovery HR (bpm). Note, it is important to have the pulse count completed in the first 20–30 seconds after the end of the 1-mile walk, and the subject should keep the legs moving to prevent pooling of blood in the periphery, which could lead to lightheadedness. The formula to calculate estimated CRF is provided in Box 7.2 (7). A modified version of this test for use in a swimming pool is also available (6).

The 1.5-mile run test requires the client to complete this distance in the shortest time possible either by running the whole distance, if possible, or by combining running with periods of walking. Ideally, the client should be able to jog for 15 minutes continuously to obtain a reasonable prediction of CRF. This test is best performed on a track and requires no other equipment.

It is important prior to either of the timed distance tests to inform the client of the purpose of the test (i.e., to estimate CRF) and emphasize that it is critical to find the best pace to cover the specific distance in the shortest amount of time possible. Effective pacing and the subject's motivation are key determinants in the outcome of this test. For many people, especially those who do not exercise regularly, finding the ideal pace takes practice. Thus, because a learning effect is likely for most people, it is ideal to perform these tests more than once to obtain a better estimate of CRF.

An estimate of $\dot{V}O_{2max}$ from the 1.5-mile run test time is derived from the following formula:

$$\dot{V}O_{2max}\,(mL \cdot kg^{-1} \cdot min^{-1}) = 3.5 + 483/1.5 \text{ mile time (min)}$$

FIXED TIME TESTS

Another variation of the 1.5-mile run test is the 12-minute walk/run test popularized by Dr. Ken Cooper of the Cooper Aerobics Clinic in Dallas, Texas. This test requires the client to cover the maximum distance in 12 minutes either by walking, running, or using a combination of both. The distance covered in 12 minutes needs to be measured and expressed in meters.

BOX 7.2	**Prediction of Cardiorespiratory Fitness from the 1-Mile Walk Test**

$$\dot{V}O_{2max} \, (mL \cdot kg^{-1} \cdot min^{-1}) = 132.853 - (0.1692 \times Wt) - (0.3877 \times Age)$$
$$+ \, (6.315 \times Gender) - (3.2649 \times Time) - (0.1565 \times HR)$$

Wt = weight in kilograms

Age = in years

Gender = 0 (women) or 1 (men)

Time = in minutes (remember to convert seconds to minutes by dividing by 60 (e.g., [42 / 60 = 0.7])

HR = recovery heart rate (HR) in bpm

EXAMPLE

A 32-year-old man who weighed 170 pounds completed the test in 12 minutes and 36 seconds with a 15-second pulse count of 35 bpm.
  Conversions:

Weight pounds to kilograms: 170 / 2.2 = 77.3 kg

Time to minutes: 12 + (36 / 60) = 12.6 min

Pulse in 15 seconds to HR: 35 × 4 = 140 bpm

$$\dot{V}O_{2max} \, (mL \cdot kg^{-1} \cdot min^{-1}) = 132.853 - (0.1692 \times 77.3) - (0.3877 \times 32)$$
$$+ \, (6.315 \times 1) - (3.2649 \times 12.6) - (0.1565$$
$$\times \, 140) = 50.6 \, mL \cdot kg^{-1} \cdot min^{-1}$$

This formula was derived on apparently healthy individuals ranging in age from 30–69 years of age (7).

The prediction of CRF from the 12-minute walk/run test is:

$$\dot{V}O_{2max} \, (mL \cdot kg^{-1} \cdot min^{-1}) = (distance \, in \, meters - 504.9) / 44.73$$

A modified version of this test for swimming is also available (3).

In clinical populations who are very deconditioned, another fixed distance test is commonly performed. The 6-minute walk test is a common procedure used as an outcome measure to evaluate progress in rehabilitation programs. Although it is considered a good indicator of functional capacity in these patients, it has generally not been a good predictor of measured $\dot{V}O_{2max}$ (8).

SUBMAXIMAL EXERCISE TESTS

A submaximal exercise test is one that requires the client to perform a fixed amount of work per unit of time. In many cases these tests require multiple stages, or levels. The key distinguishing feature of these tests is that they limit the client's effort to less than maximal exertion. There are several protocols that may be used to conduct a laboratory submaximal exercise test for the prediction of CRF using a variety of testing modalities, from the bench step, to the cycle, to the treadmill. Although some versions of step tests are done on individuals in a medical/fitness office setting, this form of administration is much less common than the use of the test within a field setting. Thus, the step test as used by groups of students is classified as a field test within this manual.

PREDICTING MAXIMAL HEART RATE

A fundamental feature of many submaximal exercise tests is the reliance on knowing the client's maximal HR value. The measurement of maximal HR requires a maximal exercise effort; thus, it cannot be obtained during submaximal exercise tests. Therefore, these submaximal testing procedures depend on the use of a prediction of maximal HR, typically estimated from age. Although there are many different prediction equations for maximal HR, most have SEE ranges of between ±10 and 15 bpm. The most commonly used equation for predicting maximal HR is:

$$\text{Age-predicted maximal HR} = 220 - \text{age (yr)}$$

These prediction equations do work well for groups. For example, if the maximal HRs of one-hundred 30-year-olds were measured, the average maximal HR for the group would be very close to 190 bpm. However, there will be approximately one in three people in this group that will have a true maximal HR of either <175 bpm or >205 bpm. This large variability in age-predicted maximal HR is one of the sources of error in predicting CRF from submaximal exercise tests. Some actual measured maximal HRs at different ages are shown in Figure 7.1 (12).

TEST TERMINATION CRITERIA

There should be clear exercise test endpoints established prior to the onset of the test. One recommendation is to use a test termination criterion of 85% of age-predicted maximal heart rate (HR_{max}). This method should result in a submaximal effort for most clients. However, it needs to be understood that those clients with actual maximal HR below (2 SEE) the age-predicted average will actually reach their actual HR_{max}. Thus, observing other signs and symptoms of maximal effort may warrant termination of the test prior to attaining the test termination criteria of 85% of age-predicted HR_{max}. Additionally, the American College of Sports Medicine (ACSM) has developed a list of indications for stopping an exercise test in adults determined to be in the low-risk stratification category, as noted in Box 7.3. As noted at the bottom of Box 7.3, there are other test termination criteria used in clinical exercise testing. These criteria will be discussed in Chapter 8, but may need to be applied in submaximal testing if the client is in the moderate- or high-risk classification.

MONITORING

As with field tests, it is important to observe the client for signs of distress and inquire about symptoms that would indicate that the test should be terminated. For the actual assessment of CRF, HR monitoring is required. As with field tests, this can be accomplished with pulse palpation or with telemetry monitoring. Because these tests are typically performed in a laboratory setting, adding blood pressure (BP) monitoring is

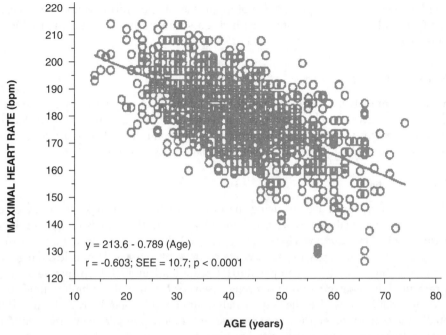

FIGURE 7.1. Variability in maximal heart rate at different ages. SEE, standard error of the estimation. (Reprinted from Whaley MH, Kaminsky LA, Dwyer GD, Getchell LH, Norton JA. Predictors of over- and underachievement of age-predicted maximal heart rate. *Med Sci Sports Exerc.* 1992;24:1173–79.)

BOX 7.3	**General Indications for Stopping an Exercise Test in Low-risk Adults[a]**

- Onset of angina or angina like symptoms
- Drop in systolic BP of >10 mmHg from baseline BP despite an increase in workload
- Excessive rise in BP: systolic pressure >250 mmHg or diastolic pressure >115 mmHg
- Shortness of breath, wheezing, leg cramps, or claudication
- Signs of poor perfusion: light-headedness, confusion, ataxia, pallor, cyanosis, nausea, or cold and clammy skin
- Failure of heart rate to increase with increased exercise intensity
- Noticeable change in heart rhythm
- Subject requests to stop
- Physical or verbal manifestations of severe fatigue
- Failure of the testing equipment

[a]Assumes that testing is nondiagnostic and is being performed without direct physician involvement or ECG monitoring. For clinical testing, Box 8–1 provides more definitive and specific termination criteria.

American College of Sports Medicine. *ACSM's Guidelines for Exercise Testing and Prescription,* 8th ed. Philadelphia (PA): Wolters Kluwer Health Ltd: , 83 p.

sometimes desired. It is important to point out that BP monitoring is not used to estimate CRF; rather, it is an optional health risk assessment to evaluate a client's BP response to exercise.

EXERCISE MODES

The most commonly used mode of exercise for submaximal exercise testing is the cycle ergometer. However, any exercise mode that allows for standardization of the work rates with known estimates of $\dot{V}O_2$ can be utilized. Both treadmills and steps are other relatively common modes of exercise for submaximal exercise testing.

Cycle Ergometer

There are several advantages to using the cycle ergometer that make it the mode of choice for submaximal exercise testing. One advantage to the cycle is the non–weight-bearing mode of exercise provided, making it a good choice for orthopedic injury cases. Also, the cycle ergometer is a relatively safe mode of exercise as there is less danger of falling off of the apparatus as compared to a treadmill. BP and HR by palpation are easily measured during exercise on the cycle ergometer because of the limited noise that the cycle produces as well as the natural stabilization of the upper body and arm. Additionally, the cycle ergometer is less expensive and is more portable than a treadmill, requires little space, and has no electrical needs.

There are a few disadvantages with the use of the cycle ergometer that merit consideration. One disadvantage is that a cycle is not a common mode of exercise or activity for many adults in the United States, especially in older populations. Another potential disadvantage is that mechanically braked cycle ergometers require the client to maintain a constant pedaling cadence to keep the work rate constant.

Generally, the mechanically braked Monark cycle ergometer is the most popular brand used for submaximal exercise testing because of the ease in calibrating the ergometer. An example of a mechanically braked cycle ergometer is shown in Figure 7.2. Calibration of this ergometer ensures accurate work outputs for the different stages of a submaximal test. The calibration procedure for the Monark cycle ergometer is provided in Box 7.4.

Proper seat height is important for optimal performance when using cycle ergometers. The knee should be flexed at approximately 5 to 10 degrees in the pedal-down position with the client seated with toes on the pedals. Figure 7.3 illustrates an incorrect seat height setting. Another way to check seat height is to have the client first place the heels on the pedals. With the heels on the pedals, the leg should be straight in the pedal-down position. Also, the seat height can be aligned with the client's greater trochanter, or hip, with the client standing next to the cycle. Most importantly, the client should actually sit on the bike, turn the pedals, and evaluate comfort with the seat height. While pedaling, the client should feel comfortable and there should be no rocking of the hips. Also, the client should maintain an upright posture, which may require an adjustment to the handlebars, and should not grip the handlebars too tightly.

Work Output Determination

Chapter 7 in *ACSM's GETP8* provides a summary of the metabolic calculation equations, which includes information on work output settings. However, because the determination of work output is a critical component of submaximal cycle exercise testing, an

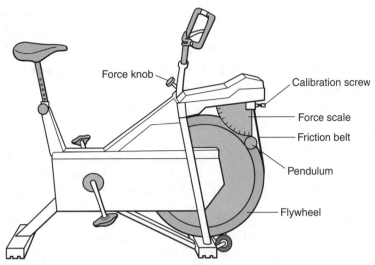

FIGURE 7.2. The features of a mechanically braked cycle ergometer. (Reprinted from Adams, G. Exercise physiology laboratory manual, 3rd ed. New York (NY): McGraw Hill: 1998, 140 p.)

BOX 7.4	**Calibration of the Monark Cycle Ergometer**

Prior to calibrating, examine the resistance belt and flywheel for excessive wear and dirt. The flywheel can be cleaned with steel wool and cleanser and the belt can also be cleaned with a mild detergent. However, you should not conduct a test if either is wet, so plan ahead. Most resistance belts have a lifespan of several years before they need replacing depending on usage.

The ergometer needs to be on a level surface for the calibration procedure.

1. Loosen or unfasten the resistance belt from the pendulum so that the pendulum hangs free. The line in the center of the pendulum should be in exact alignment with the zero line on the measurement scale. If not, loosen the lock nut to allow movement of the measurement scale to the correct zero point, and then tighten the lock screw to hold this position.
2. Using certified calibration weights (between 3 and 7 kg), hang a known weight to the balancing spring (shorter belt) and check the reading on the measurement scale. If it is not reading the exact weight, adjust the pendulum to the correct weight on the scale by means of the adjusting weight inside the pendulum. To change the position of the adjusting weight, loosen the lock screw of the weight. Should the index of the pendulum weight be too low, move the adjusting weight upward in the weight, and if the index should be too high, the adjusting weight is moved somewhat downward and locked in the new position. Repeat until the correct reading is achieved.

When the calibration is completed, reattach the belt to the mechanism and be sure to pull the belt somewhat tightly without too much slack. Check the Monark ergometer handbook[a] for more detailed information about the calibration procedures.

[a]Found at www.monark.net/eng/pdf/manual828.pdf.

overview is provided here. Work is determined by multiplying force and distance. Work output, or power, is expressed in terms of how much work is performed per unit of time. Thus, to calculate work output ($kp \cdot m \cdot min^{-1}$), the following equation is used:

$$\text{Work output} = \text{Resistance (kp)} \cdot \text{Revolutions per min (rpm)} \cdot \text{Flywheel distance (m} \cdot \text{rev}^{-1})$$

(handwritten annotation in left margin: ⑦ W.O. = 50 × 6 × resistance)

Resistance in this equation refers to the resistance caused by the flywheel by pendulum weight and friction belt and is measured in kiloponds (kp) or kilograms (kg). A kp is the force exerted by the Earth's gravity by the swinging pendulum weight applied to the friction belt on the flywheel of the cycle. Resistance can be increased during the test to apply standardized work outputs to the client. Because kp and kg are somewhat interchangeable, the measure of work on the cycle ergometer is commonly expressed as $kg \cdot m \cdot min^{-1}$.

Revolutions per minute (cadence) is simply the number of pedal revolutions per minute (rpm). Most common submaximal cycle protocols require a constant rate of 50 rpm. Newer ergometers usually have an electronic console that measures rpm; otherwise, the pedaling rate needs to be in cadence with a metronome set at 100 bpm (100 bpm for 100 downstrokes to produce 50 rpm). It is a good practice to periodically verify that the console measure is reading accurately by cross-checking it with a metronome as shown in Figure 7.4.

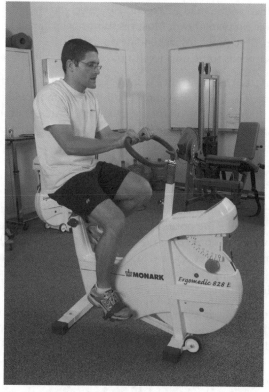

FIGURE 7.3. An example of a seat height set too low for cycle ergometry testing.

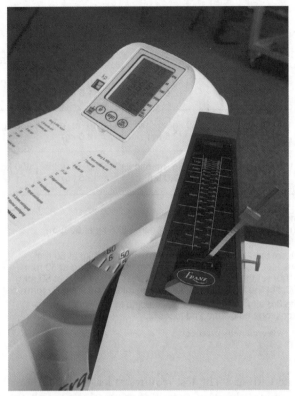

FIGURE 7.4. The use of a metronome to check the calibration of the rpm meter on a cycle.

Flywheel travel distance (meters per revolution) is a constant for each type of cycle. The Monark cycle ergometer has a 6-m · rev^{-1} ratio. This means that the flywheel on the Monark cycle will travel 6 m per complete revolution of the pedal (the flywheel is 1.62 m in circumference and travels 3.7 circuits per pedal revolution). If another brand of cycle is used, the flywheel travel distance will need to be verified.

Because the rate is standardized to 50 rpm on the Monark cycle, the client will always be covering 300 m per minute (50 rpm · 6 m · rev^{-1}). Some examples of some common cycle ergometer work output calculations using the Monark cycle at 50 rpm are as follows:

Resistance setting of 1 kg: 300 kg·m·min^{-1} = 1 kp·50 rpm·6 m·rev^{-1}

Resistance setting of 1.5 kg: 450 kg·m·min^{-1} = 1.5 kp·50 rpm·6 m·rev^{-1}

Resistance setting of 2 kg: 600 kg·m·min^{-1} = 2 kp·50 rpm·6 m·rev^{-1}

It is also important to understand another unit, called watts, used to express work output. Watts can be determined from kg · m · min^{-1} by dividing by 6.12 (usually rounded to 6). For example, 600 kg · m · min^{-1} is approximately equal to 100 watts.

YMCA SUBMAXIMAL CYCLE TEST

The protocol for the YMCA submaximal cycle test involves a branching, multistage format to gather information to establish a relationship between HR and work rate to

	1st stage	150 kg · m · min⁻¹ (0.5 kg)		
	HR <80	HR: 80-89	HR: 90-100	HR >100
2nd stage	750 kg · m · min⁻¹ (2.5 kg)	600 kg · m · min⁻¹ (2.0 kg)	450 kg · m · min⁻¹ (1.5 kg)	300 kg · m · min⁻¹ (1.0 kg)
3rd stage	900 kg · m · min⁻¹ (3.0 kg)	750 kg · m · min⁻¹ (2.5 kg)	600 kg · m · min⁻¹ (2.0 kg)	450 kg · m · min⁻¹ (1.5 kg)
4th stage	1050 kg · m · min⁻¹ (3.5 kg)	900 kg · m · min⁻¹ (3.0 kg)	700 kg · m · min⁻¹ (2.5 kg)	600 kg · m · min⁻¹ (2.0 kg)

Directions:

1 Set the 1st work rate at 150 kg · m · min⁻¹ (0.5 kg at 50 rpm)
2 If the HR in the third minute of the stage is:
   <80, set the 2nd stage at 750 kg · m · min⁻¹ (2.5 kg at 50 rpm)
   80-89, set the 2nd stage at 600 kg · m · min⁻¹ (2.0 kg at 50 rpm)
   90-100, set the 2nd stage at 450 kg · m · min⁻¹ (1.5 kg at 50 rpm)
   >100, set the 2nd stage at 300 kg · m · min⁻¹ (1.0 kg at 50 rpm)
3 Set the 3rd and 4th (if required) according to the work rates in the columns below the 2nd loads

FIGURE 7.5. YMCA cycle ergometry protocol.

ultimately estimate CRF (5). The test requires at least two and possibly four exercise stages (each of 3 minutes' duration), resulting in a total test time between 6 and 12 minutes. The requirements for the test are to complete two separate workloads that result in HR values between 110 and 150 bpm. As shown in Figure 7.5, all subjects start with a first stage workload of 150 kg · m · min⁻¹. The second stage work rate is dependent on the HR value from the first stage.

The recommended procedures for this test are provided in Box 7.5. It is important to ensure that the client maintains a pedal rate of 50 (±2) rpm throughout the test. At each 3-minute work stage, a steady-state HR is required, which is operationally defined as a HR at the end of the second and third minute of each stage that does not increase more than 5 bpm. If the HR has increased more than 5 bpm, this indicates that the client has not reached steady state and the stage should be continued for another minute. The resistance setting of the cycle ergometer (provided by the measurement scale on the side of the ergometer) and the pedal rate (50 rpm) should be checked regularly throughout the test and corrected if necessary. Although exercise BP measurements are not required for the computation of CRF, it is suggested that they be taken and recorded at each stage. These data would be used to end a test early in the event a client has a hypertensive response. Further, if the client does in fact have a significantly elevated BP during the test, these data could be valuable for the client's healthcare professional.

Estimating $\dot{V}O_{2max}$

There are two methods that can be used to derive an estimate of CRF. One involves plotting the data on a graph and using an extrapolation technique, and the other uses a calculation-based formula.

BOX 7.5	General Procedures for Submaximal Testing of Cardiorespiratory Fitness

1. Obtain resting heart rate and BP immediately before exercise in the exercise posture.
2. The client should be familiarized with the ergometer. If using a cycle ergometer, properly position the client on the ergometer (i.e., upright posture, five-degree bend in the knee at maximal leg extension, hands in proper position on handlebars).
3. The exercise test should begin with a two- to three-minute warm-up to acquaint the client with the cycle ergometer and prepare him or her for the exercise intensity in the first stage of the test.
4. A specific protocol should consist of 2- or 3-minute stages with appropriate increments in work rate.
5. Heart rate should be monitored at least two times during each stage, near the end of the second and third minutes of each stage. If heart rate >110 beats $\cdot$ min^{-1}, steady-state heart rate (i.e., two heart rates within 5 beats $\cdot$ min^{-1}) should be reached before the workload is increased.
6. Blood pressure should be monitored in the last minute of each stage and repeated (verified) in the event of a hypotensive or hypertensive response.
7. Perceived exertion and additional rating scales should be monitored near the end of the last minute of each stage using either the 6–20 or 0–10 scale (*GETP8* Table 4.7).
8. Client appearance and symptoms should be monitored and recorded regularly.
9. The test should be terminated when the subject reaches 70% heart rate reserve (85% of age-predicted maximal heart rate), fails to conform to the exercise test protocol, experiences adverse signs or symptoms, requests to stop, or experiences an emergency situation.
10. An appropriate cool-down/recovery period should be initiated consisting of either:
    a. Continued exercise at a work rate equivalent to that of the first stage of the exercise test protocol or lower; or
    b. A passive cool-down if the subject experiences signs of discomfort or an emergency situation occurs
11. All physiologic observations (e.g., heart rate, BP, signs and symptoms) should be continued for at least 5 minutes of recovery unless abnormal responses occur, which would warrant a longer posttest surveillance period. Continue low-level exercise until heart rate and BP stabilize, but not necessarily until they reach pre-exercise levels.

From American College of Sports Medicine. *ACSM's Guidelines for Exercise Testing and Prescription*, 8th ed. Philadelphia (PA): Wolters Kluwer Health Ltd: 2009, 81 p.

Graphing Technique

The graphing method requires that the two HR and work output data points be plotted on a graph like the one provided in Figure 7.6. A horizontal line is drawn across the graph to intersect the y-axis (HR) at the value of age-predicted maximal HR. Then a straight line connecting the two data points is drawn. This line is extended

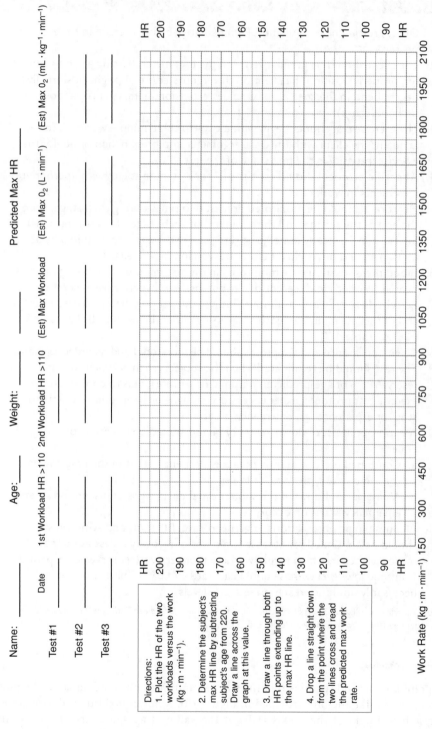

Name: _____

Age: _____   Weight: _____   Predicted Max HR _____

	Date	1st Workload HR >110	2nd Workload HR >110	(Est) Max Workload	(Est) Max O$_2$ (L · min^{-1})	(Est) Max O$_2$ (mL · kg^{-1} · min^{-1})
Test #1	_____	_____	_____	_____	_____	_____
Test #2	_____	_____	_____	_____	_____	_____
Test #3	_____	_____	_____	_____	_____	_____

Directions:
1. Plot the HR of the two workloads versus the work (kg · m · min^{-1}).

2. Determine the subject's max HR line by subtracting subject's age from 220. Draw a line across the graph at this value.

3. Draw a line through both HR points extending up to the max HR line.

4. Drop a line straight down from the point where the two lines cross and read the predicted max work rate.

Work Rate (kg · m · min^{-1})

FIGURE 7.6. A graph used for the prediction of $\dot{V}O_{2max}$ from cycle ergometry tests.

124

(extrapolated) up to the horizontal line. Finally, a perpendicular line is drawn down from this point of intersection to the x-axis (work rate). This work rate value is the predicted maximal work rate and is used in the ACSM metabolic equation for leg cycling to calculate a predicted $\dot{V}O_{2max}$.

$$\dot{V}O_2 \,(\text{mL·kg}^{-1}\text{·min}^{-1}) = [(1.8 \times \text{work rate}) / \text{Body wt in kg}] + 7$$

Figure 7.7 demonstrates the process of graphing the HR response for prediction of $\dot{V}O_{2max}$. This figure also contains an example of how the inaccuracy of age-predicted maximal HR might influence the results.

Calculation-based Formula

To calculate a predicted $\dot{V}O_{2max}$, it is necessary to first calculate the slope of the HR and $\dot{V}O_2$ relationship. The slope (m) will then be used within a standard linear regression equation of the form y = mx + b, where the y variable represents $\dot{V}O_2$ and where the the x variable represents HR.

Calculation of slope:

$$\text{Slope (m)} = (\dot{V}O_2 2 - \dot{V}O_2 1)/(HR2 - HR1)$$

where

$$\dot{V}O_2 1 = \text{Submaximal predicted } \dot{V}O_2 \text{ from stage 1, in mL} \cdot \text{kg}^{-1} \cdot \text{min}^{-1}$$

$$\dot{V}O_2 2 = \text{Submaximal predicted } \dot{V}O_2 \text{ from stage 2, in mL} \cdot \text{kg}^{-1} \cdot \text{min}^{-1}$$

$$HR1 = \text{HR from stage 1, in bpm}$$

$$HR2 = \text{HR from stage 2, in bpm}$$

$\dot{V}O_{2max}$ is then estimated from the following equation:

$$\dot{V}O_{2max} \,(\text{in mL·kg}^{-1}\text{·min}^{-1}) = m \,(HR_{max} - HR2) + \dot{V}O_2 2$$

where

$$HR_{max} = 220 - \text{age}$$

For example, a 30-year-old male (75 kg) completed two stages (450 and 600 kg · m · min^{-1}) with HR values of 116 and 130 bpm, respectively. His $\dot{V}O_{2max}$ would be calculated as follows:

$$\dot{V}O_2 1 \,(\text{mL·kg}^{-1}\text{·min}^{-1}) = [(1.8 \times \text{work rate})/\text{Body wt in kg}] + 7$$

$$= [(1.8 \times 450)/75] + 7 = 17.8$$

$$\dot{V}O_2 2 \,(\text{mL·kg}^{-1}\text{·min}^{-1}) = [(1.8 \times \text{work rate})/\text{Body wt in kg}] + 7$$

$$= [(1.8 \times 600)/75] + 7 = 21.4$$

$$m = (21.4 - 17.8)\,(130 - 116) = 0.257$$

$$\dot{V}O_{2max} \,(\text{mL·kg}^{-1}\text{·min}^{-1}) = m \,(HR_{max} - HR2) + \dot{V}O_2 2$$

$$= [0.257\,((220 - 30) - 130)] + 21.4$$

$$= 36.8 \text{ mL·kg}^{-1}\text{·min}^{-1}$$

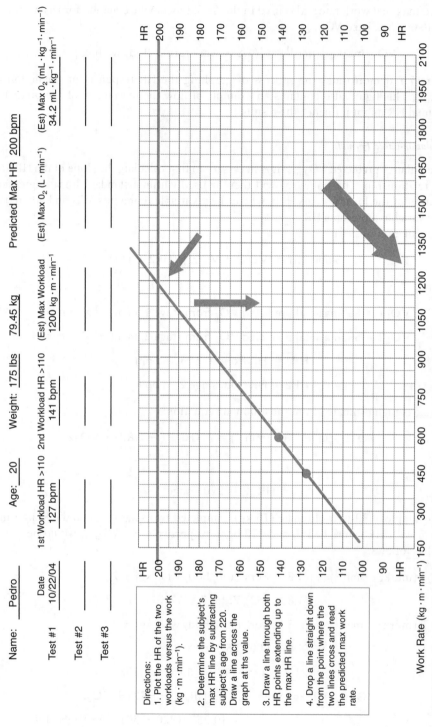

Name: Pedro Date 10/22/04 Age: 20 Weight: 175 lbs 1st Workload HR >110 127 bpm 2nd Workload HR >110 141 bpm 79.45 kg (Est) Max Workload 1200 kg · m · min⁻¹ Predicted Max HR 200 bpm (Est) Max O₂ (L · min⁻¹) (Est) Max O₂ (mL · kg⁻¹ · min⁻¹) 34.2 mL · kg⁻¹ · min⁻¹

Test #1
Test #2
Test #3

Directions:
1. Plot the HR of the two workloads versus the work (kg · m · min⁻¹).

2. Determine the subject's max HR line by subtracting subject's age from 220. Draw a line across the graph at ths value.

3. Draw a line through both HR points extending up to the max HR line.

4. Drop a line straight down from the point where the two lines cross and read the predicted max work rate.

Work Rate (kg · m · min⁻¹)

FIGURE 7.7. Description of the process of graphing the heart rate response for prediction of $\dot{V}O_{2max}$.

TABLE 7.1. ÅSTRAND CYCLE SUBMAXIMAL CYCLE ERGOMETER TEST INITIAL WORKLOADS

This protocol table is designed as a guide. The protocol is designed to elicit an HR of between 125–170 bpm by 6 minutes. You can adjust the work output as necessary during the test (usually after the first 6 minutes) to achieve an HR in or near this range in your subject.

INDIVIDUAL	WORK OUTPUT ($kp \cdot m^{-1} \cdot min^{-1}$)
Men	
Unconditioned	300–600
Conditioned	600–900
Women	
Unconditioned	300–450
Conditioned	450–600
Poorly Conditioned or Older Individuals	300

ÅSTRAND SUBMAXIMAL CYCLE ERGOMETER TEST

Per Olaf Åstrand (a noted exercise physiologist from Sweden), along with his wife, Irma Ryhming, developed a simple protocol in the 1950s to predict CRF from laboratory submaximal cycle exercise results. This protocol is sometimes known as the Åstrand-Ryhming protocol. The client typically performs one 6-minute submaximal exercise stage of a standardized work rate. The work rate is selected according to recommendations found in Table 7.1. This procedure requires an exercise HR value between 125 and 170 bpm. Most of the procedures are similar to the YMCA protocol including maintaining a 50 rpm pedal rate and monitoring the client throughout the test. A steady-state HR is required at the end of the 6-minute work stage. If the HR is below 125 bpm, then workload is increased and the test continues for an additional 6 minutes, making the total test time range the same as for the YMCA protocol.

Estimating $\dot{V}O_{2max}$

There are two methods that can be used to derive an estimate of CRF. One involves plotting the data on a graph called a nomogram, and the other uses a calculation-based formula.

Nomogram Technique

A nomogram is a graphic representation where two known data points are plotted and connected with a line to predict a third, unknown value. Figure 7.8 depicts a nomogram used for calculating the unknown $\dot{V}O_{2max}$ from the pulse rate during submaximal work (11). Using this nomogram technique, a mark is placed on the pulse rate scale (left side of nomogram) at the steady-state HR (value must be between 125 and 170 bpm). Note that this scale actually has two sides, one for men (left) and one for women (right). Next, a mark is placed on the workload scale (right side of nomogram). Note that this scale also has two sides, one for men (right) and one for women (left). The two points are connected with a straight line and the $\dot{V}O_{2max}$ is read from the center scale. The correction factor table found in Table 7.2 must then be used to adjust the $\dot{V}O_{2max}$ for the person's age (nearest 5 years). For example, if the $\dot{V}O_{2max}$ was estimated to be $3.65 \text{ L} \cdot min^{-1}$ from the nomogram, the corrected value for a 40-year-old man would be $3.03 \text{ L} \cdot min^{-1}$ (3.65×0.83).

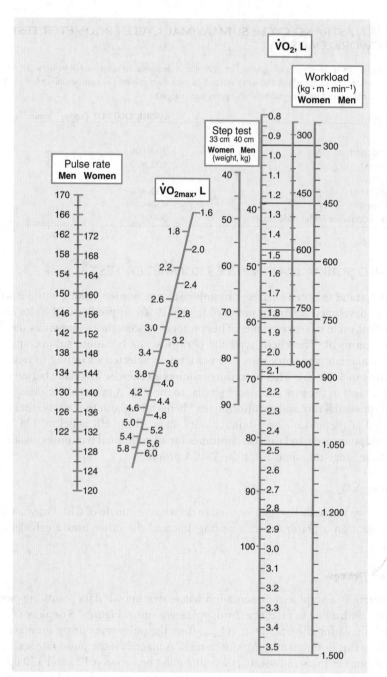

FIGURE 7.8. Modified Åstrand-Ryhming nomogram. (From Astrand P-O, Ryhming I. A nomogram for calculation of aerobic capacity [physical fitness] from pulse rate during submaximal work. *J Appl Physiol* 1954;7:218–221, with permission.)

TABLE 7.2. AGE CORRECTION FACTOR FOR ÅSTRAND CYCLE ERGOMETER TEST RESULTS

AGE	CORRECTION FACTOR
15	1.10
25	1.00
35	0.87
40	0.83
45	0.78
50	0.75
55	0.71
60	0.68
65	0.65

Adapted from *ACSM's Health-Related Physical Fitness Assessment Manual,* 2nd ed. Philadelphia (PA): Wolters Kluwer Health Ltd: 2005, 121 p.

Calculation-based Formula

To calculate the $\dot{V}O_{2max}$, in $mL \cdot kg^{-1} \cdot min^{-1}$ from the single-stage Åstrand protocol, the following formula is utilized:

$$\dot{V}O_{2max} (mL \cdot kg^{-1} \cdot min^{-1})$$
$$= \dot{V}O_2 1 \left[(220 - age - 73 - (G \times 10))/(HR - 73 - (G \times 10)) \right]$$

where

$$\dot{V}O_2 1 = \text{submaximal workload } (\dot{V}O_2, \text{ in } (mL \cdot kg^{-1} \cdot min^{-1}))$$

$$G = 0 \text{ for women and 1 for men}$$

$$HR = \text{steady-state HR, in bpm}$$

For example, calculate $\dot{V}O_{2max}$ for a 33-year-old conditioned woman (63 kg), with a single stage of $600 \ kg \cdot m \cdot min^{-1}$ where the HR value was 124 bpm, as follows:

Solve for $\dot{V}O_2 1$:

$$\dot{V}O_2 1 (mL \cdot kg^{-1} \cdot min^{-1}) = \left[(1.8 \times \text{work rate})/\text{Body wt in kg} \right] + 7$$
$$= \left[(1.8 \times 600)/63 \right] + 7 = 24.1$$

Then, insert $\dot{V}O_2 1$ and appropriate gender, age, and HR values into formula:

$$\dot{V}O_{2max} (mL \cdot kg^{-1} \cdot min^{-1})$$
$$= \dot{V}O_2 1 \left[(220 - age - 73 - (G \times 10))/(HR - 73 - (G \times 10)) \right]$$
$$= 24.1 \left[(220 - 33 - 73 - (0 \times 10))/(124 - 73 - (0 \times 10)) \right]$$
$$= 53.8 \ mL \cdot kg^{-1} \cdot min^{-1}$$

TREADMILL

A submaximal treadmill exercise test can also be used to predict CRF. Thus, the same basic principle as used for the YMCA cycle test, namely determining the specific linear relationship between HR and $\dot{V}O_2$, is used to derive the estimate. The same HR range of two work stages with HR values between 110 and 150 bpm is recommended.

Although there are many different treadmill protocols, as will be discussed in Chapter 8, a common one used for submaximal assessments is the Bruce protocol. Most clients should be able to obtain two HR values between 110 and 150 bpm within the first three stages (each 3 minutes in duration) of this protocol. (Note: the entire protocol is found in Chapter 8, Table 8.3.)

The basic procedures are identical to the YMCA submaximal cycle protocol with the exception of the mode of exercise. The warm-up minute is performed at 1.7 mph with no elevation. If the client's HR is ≥ 110 bpm at the first stage, then only one additional stage is required. Thus, this test will last between 6 and 9 minutes.

TABLE 7.3. PERCENTILE VALUES FOR MAXIMAL AEROBIC POWER (MALES)

		MALES							
		AGE 20–29				AGE 30–39			
%	BALKE TREADMILL (time)	MAX $\dot{V}O_2$ (mL/kg/min)	12 MIN RUN (miles)	1.5 MILE RUN (time)	BALKE TREADMILL (time)	MAX $\dot{V}O_2$ (mL/kg/min)	12 MIN RUN (miles)	1.5 MILE RUN (time)	
99	32:00	61.2	2.02	8:22	30:00	58.3	1.94	8:49	
95	28:31	56.2	1.88	9:10	27:11	54.3	1.82	9:31	S
90	27:00	54.0	1.81	9:34	26:00	52.5	1.77	9:52	
85	26:00	52.5	1.77	9:52	24:45	50.7	1.72	10:14	
80	25:00	51.1	1.73	10:08	23:30	47.5	1.67	10:38	E
75	23:40	49.2	1.68	10:34	22:30	47.5	1.63	10:59	
70	23:00	48.2	1.65	10:49	22:00	46.8	1.61	11.09	
65	22:00	46.8	1.61	11:09	21:00	45.3	1.57	11:34	
60	21:15	45.7	1.58	11:27	20:20	44.4	1.55	11:49	G
55	21:00	45.3	1.57	11:34	20:00	43.9	1.53	11:58	
50	20:00	43.9	1.53	11:58	19:00	42.4	1:49	12:25	
45	19:26	43.1	1.51	12:11	18:15	41.4	1.46	12:44	
40	18:50	42.2	1.49	12:29	18:00	41.0	1.45	12:53	F
35	18:00	41.0	1.45	12:53	17:00	39.5	1.41	13:25	
30	17:30	40.3	1.43	13:08	16:15	38.5	1.38	13:48	
25	17:00	39.5	1.41	13:25	15:40	37.6	1.36	14:10	
20	16:00	38.1	1.37	13:58	15:00	36.7	1.33	14:33	P
15	15:00	36.7	1.33	14:33	14:00	35.2	1.29	15:14	
10	14:00	35.2	1.29	15:14	13:00	33.8	1.25	15:56	
5	12:00	32.3	1.21	16:46	11:10	31.1	1.18	17:30	
1	8:00	26:6	1.05	20:55	8:00	26.6	1.05	20:55	VP
	n = 2,606				n = 13,158				

Total n = 15,764

S, superior; E, excellent; G, good; F, fair; P, poor; VP, very poor.

From American College of Sports Medicine. *ACSM's Guidelines for Exercise Testing and Prescription*, 8th ed. Philadelphia (PA): Wolters Kluwer Health Ltd: 2009, 84-86 pp.

TABLE 7.3. PERCENTILE VALUES FOR MAXIMAL AEROBIC POWER (MALES) (*Continued*)

MALES

	AGE 40–49				AGE 50–59				
%	**BALKE TREADMILL (time)**	**MAX $\dot{V}O_2$ (mL/kg/ min)**	**12 MIN RUN (miles)**	**1.5 MILE RUN (time)**	**BALKE TREADMILL (time)**	**MAX $\dot{V}O_2$ (mL/kg/ min)**	**12 MIN RUN (miles)**	**1.5 MILE RUN (time)**	
99	29:06	57.0	1.90	9:02	27:15	54.3	1.82	9:31	
95	26:16	52.9	1.79	9:47	24:00	49.7	1.69	10:27	S
90	25:00	51.1	1.73	10:09	22:00	46.8	1.61	11:09	
85	23:14	48.5	1.66	10:44	20:31	44.6	1.55	11:45	
80	22:00	46.8	1.61	11:09	19:35	43.3	1.52	12:08	E
75	21:02	45.4	1.58	11:32	18:32	41.8	1.47	12:37	
70	20:15	44.2	1.54	11:52	18:00	41.0	1.45	12:53	
65	20:00	43.9	1.53	11:58	17:00	39.5	1.41	13:25	
60	19:00	42.4	1.49	12:25	16:10	38.3	1.38	13.53	G
55	18:02	41.0	1.45	12:53	16:00	38.1	1.37	13:58	
50	17:34	40.4	1.44	13:05	15:02	36.7	1.33	14:33	
45	17:00	39.5	1.41	13:25	14:56	36.6	1.33	14:35	
40	16:12	38.4	1.38	13:50	14:00	35.2	1.29	15:14	F
35	15:38	37.6	1.36	14:10	13:05	33.9	1.26	15:53	
30	15:00	36.7	1.33	14:33	12:38	33.2	1.24	16:16	
25	14:20	35.7	1.31	15:00	12:00	32.3	1.21	16:46	
20	13:35	34.6	1.28	15:32	11:10	31.1	1.18	17:30	P
15	12:45	33.4	1.24	16:09	10:15	29.8	1.14	18:22	
10	11:40	31.8	1.20	17:04	9:15	28.4	1.10	19:24	
5	10:00	29.4	1.13	18:39	7:30	25.8	1.03	21:40	
1	7:00	25.1	1.01	22.22	4:20	21.3	0.90	27:08	VP
	n = 16,534				n = 9,102				

Total n = 25,636

S, superior; E, excellent; G, good; F, fair; P, poor; VP, very poor.

From American College of Sports Medicine. *ACSM's Guidelines for Exercise Testing and Prescription,* 8th ed. Philadelphia (PA): Wolters Kluwer Health Ltd: 2009, 84-86 pp.

Estimating $\dot{V}O_{2max}$

$\dot{V}O_{2max}$ is then estimated from the same equation that was used with the YMCA cycle protocol:

$$\dot{V}O_{2max} \text{ (in mL} \cdot \text{kg}^{-1} \cdot \text{min}^{-1}) = m \, (HR_{max} - HR2) + \dot{V}O_2 2$$

However, the work rate value is now derived from speed (S) and grade (G) on the treadmill and is used in the ACSM metabolic equation to calculate a predicted $\dot{V}O_2$.

$$\dot{V}O_2 \text{ (mL} \cdot \text{kg}^{-1} \cdot \text{min}^{-1}) = [(0.1 \times S) + (1.8 \times S \times G) + 3.5$$

where

$$S \text{ (speed)} = \text{mph} \times 26.8 \text{ m} \cdot \text{min}^{-1} \cdot \text{mph}^{-1}$$

$$G \text{ (grade)} = \% \text{ elevation} / 100$$

TABLE 7.3. PERCENTILE VALUES FOR MAXIMAL AEROBIC POWER (MALES) (*Continued*)

	MALES								
	AGE 60–69				**AGE 70–79**				
%	**BALKE TREADMILL (time)**	**MAX $\dot{V}O_2$ (mL/kg/min)**	**12 MIN RUN (miles)**	**1.5 MILE RUN (time)**	**BALKE TREADMILL (time)**	**MAX $\dot{V}O_2$ (mL/kg/min)**	**12 MIN RUN (miles)**	**1.5 MILE RUN (time)**	
99	25:02	51.1	1.74	10:09	24:00	49.7	1.69	10:27	
95	21:33	46.1	1.60	11:20	19:00	42.4	1.49	12:25	S
90	19:30	43.2	1.51	12:10	17:00	39.5	1.41	13:25	
85	18:00	41.0	1.45	12:53	16:00	38.1	1.37	13:57	
80	17:00	39.5	1.41	13:25	14:34	36.0	1.32	14:52	E
75	16:00	38.1	1.37	13:58	13:25	34.4	1.27	15:38	
70	15:00	36.7	1.33	14:33	12:27	33.0	1.23	16:22	
65	14:30	35.9	1.31	14:55	12:00	32.3	1.21	16:46	
60	13:51	35.0	1.29	15:20	11:00	30.9	1.17	17:37	G
55	13:04	33.9	1.26	15:53	10:30	30.2	1.15	18:05	
50	12:30	33.1	1.23	16:19	10:00	29.4	1.13	18:39	
45	12:00	32.3	1.21	16:46	9:20	28.5	1.11	19:19	
40	11:21	31.4	1.19	17:19	9:00	28.0	1.09	19:43	F
35	10:49	30.6	1.17	17:49	8:21	27.1	1.07	20:28	
30	10:00	29.4	1.13	18:39	7:38	26.0	1.04	21:28	
25	9:29	28.7	1.11	19:10	7:00	25.1	1.01	22:22	
20	8:37	27.4	1.08	20:13	6:00	23.7	0.97	23:55	P
15	7:33	25.9	1.03	21:34	5:00	22.2	0.93	25:49	
10	6:20	24.1	0.99	23:27	4:00	20.8	0.89	27:55	
5	4:55	22.1	0.93	25:58	3:00	19.3	0.85	30:34	
1	2:29	18.6	0.83	31:59	2:00	17.9	0.81	33:30	VP
		n = 2,682				n = 467			

Total n = 3,149

S, superior; E, excellent; G, good; F, fair; P, poor; VP, very poor.

From American College of Sports Medicine. *ACSM's Guidelines for Exercise Testing and Prescription,* 8th ed. Philadelphia (PA): Wolters Kluwer Health Ltd: 2009, 84-86 pp.

For example, the first stage with a speed of 1.7 mph and a grade of 10% would have a predicted $\dot{V}O_2$ for this stage calculated as follows:

$$\dot{V}O_2 \, (\text{mL} \cdot \text{kg}^{-1} \cdot \text{min}^{-1}) = [(0.1 \times [1.7 \times 26.8]) + (1.8 \times [1.7 \times 26.8]$$
$$\times [10 / 100]) + 3.5$$
$$= 16.2 \, \text{mL} \cdot \text{kg}^{-1} \cdot \text{min}^{-1}$$

INTERPRETATION

Normative standards for CRF have not been developed. The ACSM has used the reference values established by the Cooper Institute, which are shown in Tables 7.3 and 7.4 for interpretation. It is important to recognize that these values are based on the population that has received these measures and are expressed as percentiles, which may limit their usefulness for interpreting test results from populations with different characteristics.

TABLE 7.4. PERCENTILE VALUES FOR MAXIMAL AEROBIC POWER (FEMALES)

	FEMALES								
	AGE 20–29				AGE 30–39				
%	BALKE TREADMILL (time)	MAX $\dot{V}O_2$ (mL/kg/ min)	12 MIN RUN (miles)	1.5 MILE RUN (time)	BALKE TREADMILL (time)	MAX $\dot{V}O_2$ (mL/kg/ min)	12 MIN RUN (miles)	1.5 MILE RUN (time)	
99	27:43	55.0	1.84	9:23	26:00	52.5	1.77	9:52	
95	24:24	50.2	1.71	10:20	22:06	46.9	1.62	11:08	S
90	22:30	47.5	1.63	10:59	20:34	44.7	1.56	11:43	
85	21:00	45.3	1.57	11:34	19:03	42.5	1.50	12:23	
80	20:04	44.0	1.54	11:56	18:00	41.0	1.45	12:53	E
75	19:42	43.4	1.52	12:07	17:30	40.3	1.43	13:08	
70	18:06	41.1	1.46	12:51	16:30	38.8	1.39	13:41	
65	17:45	40.6	1.44	13:01	16:00	38.1	1.37	13.58	
60	17:00	39.5	1.41	13:25	15:02	36.7	1.33	14:33	G
55	16:00	38.1	1.37	13:58	15:00	36.7	1.33	14:33	
50	15:30	37.4	1.35	14:15	14:00	35.2	1.29	15:14	
45	15:00	36.7	1.33	14:33	13:30	34.5	1.27	15:35	
40	14:11	35.5	1.30	15:05	13:00	33.8	1.25	15:56	F
35	13:36	34.6	1.27	15:32	12:03	32.4	1.21	16:43	
30	13:00	33.8	1.25	15:56	12:00	32.3	1.21	16:46	
25	12:04	32.4	1.22	16:43	11:00	30.9	1.17	17:38	
20	11:30	31.6	1.19	17:11	10:20	29.9	1.15	18:18	P
15	10:42	30.5	1.16	17:53	9:39	28.9	1.12	19:01	
10	10:00	29.4	1.13	18:39	8:36	27.4	1.08	20:13	
5	7:54	26.4	1.05	21:05	7:16	25.5	1.02	21:57	
1	5:14	22.6	0.94	25:17	5:20	22.7	0.94	25:10	VP
	n = 1,350				n = 4,394				
Total n = 5,744									

S, superior; E, excellent; G, good; F, fair; P, poor; VP, very poor.

From American College of Sports Medicine. *ACSM's Guidelines for Exercise Testing and Prescription,* 8th ed. Philadelphia (PA): Wolters Kluwer Health Ltd: 2009, 87-89 pp.

As indicated earlier in this chapter, the gold standard test for CRF is a maximal exercise test with $\dot{V}O_{2max}$ measured from the collection of expired gases. Because both field tests and submaximal exercise tests require prediction of $\dot{V}O_{2max}$, the interpretation of the results need to include an expression of SEE. Unfortunately, some of the prediction equations used do not provide an SEE.

SOURCES OF ERROR IN SUBMAXIMAL PREDICTION

There are several potential sources of error in submaximal exercise tests when predicting $\dot{V}O_{2max}$. Certainly, any errors in the measurement of workload (this would include using an ergometer that was not properly calibrated) or in the measurement of HR will result in prediction error.

One primary source of error is that associated with age-predicted maximal HR. This variability between individuals was covered earlier and an example of the potential for error can be observed using Figure 7.7 by observing the difference in predicted maximal work rate if the actual maximal heart rate was 180 bpm.

TABLE 7.4. PERCENTILE VALUES FOR MAXIMAL AEROBIC POWER (FEMALES) (*Continued*)

		FEMALES							
		AGE 40–49				AGE 50–59			
%	BALKE TREADMILL (time)	MAX V̇O₂ (mL/kg/ min)	12 MIN RUN (miles)	1.5 MILE RUN (time)	BALKE TREADMILL (time)	MAX V̇O₂ (mL/kg/ min)	12 MIN RUN (miles)	1.5 MILE RUN (time)	
99	25:00	51.1	1.74	10:09	21:00	45.3	1.57	11:34	
95	20:56	45.2	1.57	11:35	17:16	39.9	1.42	13:16	S
90	19:00	42.4	1.49	12:25	16:00	38.1	1.37	13:58	
85	17:20	40.0	1.43	13:14	15:00	36.7	1.33	14:33	
80	16:34	38.9	1.40	13:38	14:00	35.2	1.29	15:14	E
75	16:00	38.1	1.37	13:58	13:15	34.1	1.26	15:47	
70	15:00	36.7	1.33	14:33	12:23	32.9	1.23	16:26	
65	14:14	35.6	1.30	15:03	12:00	32.3	1.21	16:46	
60	13:56	35.1	1.29	15:17	11:23	31.4	1.19	17:19	G
55	13:02	33.8	1.25	15:56	11:00	30.9	1.17	17:38	
50	12:39	33.3	1.24	16:13	10:30	30.2	1.15	18:05	
45	12:00	32.3	1.21	16:46	10:00	29.4	1.13	18:39	
40	11:30	31.6	1.19	17:11	9:30	28.7	1.11	19:10	F
35	11:00	30.9	1.17	17:38	9:00	28.0	1.09	19:43	
30	10:10	29.7	1.14	18:26	8:30	27.3	1.07	20:17	
25	10:00	29.4	1.13	18:39	8:00	26.6	1.05	20:55	
20	9:00	28.0	1.09	19:43	7:15	25.5	1.02	21:57	P
15	8:07	26.7	1.06	20:49	6:40	24.6	1.00	22:53	
10	7:21	25.6	1.03	21:52	6:00	23.7	0.97	23:55	
5	6:17	24.1	0.98	23:27	4:48	21.9	0.92	26:15	
1	4:00	20.8	0.89	27:55	3:00	19.3	0.85	30:34	VP
	n = 4,834				n = 3,103				
Total n = 7,937									

S, superior; E, excellent; G, good; F, fair; P, poor; VP, very poor.

From American College of Sports Medicine. *ACSM's Guidelines for Exercise Testing and Prescription*, 8th ed. Philadelphia (PA): Wolters Kluwer Health Ltd: 2009, 87-89 pp.

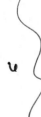

A second source of error is the variability in mechanical efficiency on an ergometer. In other words, some people will be more efficient (meaning they will require less O_2 to perform a given work rate). The *GETP7e* states, "The intersubject variability in measured V̇O₂ may have a standard error of estimate as high as 7% for performing a given work rate."

A third source of error is the variability in submaximal HR at the same work rate on different days. One study by Davies (4) reported that at intensities producing HR between 120 and 150 bpm, the HR varied by ±8% on different days. This is notable because this is the recommended HR range for the YMCA cycle ergometer protocol.

The final source of error is the possibility of a break in linearity of HR and V̇O₂ as the values approach maximum. Some individuals may have larger increases in V̇O₂ compared to the increase in HR as they approach maximum.

Any and all of these factors may be involved in any submaximal exercise test. The reported SEE range for these types of tests ranges between ±10% and ±20%.

TABLE 7.4. PERCENTILE VALUES FOR MAXIMAL AEROBIC POWER (FEMALES) (*Continued*)

	FEMALES								
	AGE 60–69				AGE 70–79				
%	BALKE TREADMILL (time)	MAX $\dot{V}O_2$ (mL/kg/min)	12 MIN RUN (miles)	1.5 MILE RUN (time)	BALKE TREADMILL (time)	MAX $\dot{V}O_2$ (mL/kg/min)	12 MIN RUN (miles)	1.5 MILE RUN (time)	
99	19:00	42.4	1.49	12:25	19:00	42.4	1.49	12:25	
95	15:09	36.9	1.34	14:28	15:00	36.7	1.33	14:33	S
90	13:33	34.6	1.27	15:32	12:50	33.5	1.25	16:06	
85	12:28	33.0	1.23	16:22	11:46	32.0	1.20	16:57	
80	12:00	32.3	1.21	16:46	10:30	30.2	1.15	18:05	E
75	11:04	31.0	1.18	17:34	10:00	29.4	1.13	18:39	
70	10:30	30.2	1.15	18:05	9:15	28.4	1.10	19:24	
65	10:00	29.4	1.13	18:39	8:43	27.6	1.08	20:02	
60	9:44	29.1	1.12	18:52	8:00	26.6	1.05	20:54	G
55	9:11	28.3	1.10	19:29	7:37	26.0	1.04	21:45	
50	8:40	27.5	1.08	20:08	7:00	25.1	1.01	22:22	
45	8:15	26.9	1.06	20:38	6:39	24.6	1.00	22:54	
40	8:00	26.6	1.05	20:55	6:05	23.8	0.98	23:47	F
35	7:14	25.4	1.02	22:03	5:28	22.9	0.95	24:54	
30	6:52	24.9	1.01	22:34	5:00	22.2	0.93	25:49	
25	6:21	24.2	0.99	23:20	4:45	21.9	0.92	26:15	
20	6:00	23.7	0.97	23:55	4:16	21.2	0.90	27:17	P
15	5:25	22.8	0.95	25:02	4:00	20.8	0.89	27:55	
10	4:40	21.7	0.92	26:32	3:00	19.3	0.85	30:34	
5	3:30	20.1	0.87	29:06	2:00	17.9	0.81	33:32	
1	2:10	18.1	0.82	33:05	1:00	16.4	0.77	37:26	VP
	n = 1,088				n = 209				

Total n = 1,297

S, superior; E, excellent; G, good; F, fair; P, poor; VP, very poor.

From American College of Sports Medicine. *ACSM's Guidelines for Exercise Testing and Prescription*, 8th ed. Philadelphia (PA): Wolters Kluwer Health Ltd: 2009, 87-89 pp.

SUMMARY

CRF is an important component of health-related physical fitness and one that is commonly desired by clients. Because the measurement of $\dot{V}O_{2max}$ is limited by factors such as the time required, the cost, and the availability, field tests and submaximal exercise tests are frequently performed. As with other measures obtained via prediction equations, appropriate care is needed in interpreting the results of these CRF prediction methods.

> > > LABORATORY ACTIVITIES

FIELD TEST ASSESSMENTS OF CARDIORESPIRATORY FITNESS

Data Collection
Form groups of three. Each person is required to do the Queens College step test and one of the following field tests to estimate CRF: 1.5-mile run, 12-minute run/walk, or 1-mile walk. Follow the instructions for each test provided in this chapter.

Laboratory Report
1. Provide the data collected for each test in a summary table along with calculations to estimate CRF from the two field tests.
2. Provide an interpretation (classification according to Table 7.3 or 7.4) of your estimated VO_{2max}.
3. Discuss possible reasons for the differences in CRF estimates between tests.

SUBMAXIMAL EXERCISE TEST ASSESSMENTS OF CARDIORESPIRATORY FITNESS

Data Collection
Form groups of three. One person in the group will do the YMCA cycle test, one person will do the Åstrand-Ryhming cycle, and one person will do the Bruce test. Follow the instructions for each test provided in this chapter.

Laboratory Report
1. Provide the data collected for each test in a summary table along with calculations to estimate CRF from the three tests. Note: you need to perform both the graphing method and the calculation methods to estimate VO_{2max}.
2. Provide an interpretation (classification according to Table 7.3 or 7.4) of your estimated VO_{2max}.
3. Discuss possible reasons for the differences in CRF estimates between this test and the field tests you performed in the previous lab.
4. Which of the above tests do you feel best estimates your fitness level and why?

> > > CASE STUDY

Molly is a 28-year-old business woman who has decided after years of being irregularly active to "get back in shape." Molly ran track in high school and remembers doing the 1.5-mile run test in college. She decides to head to the track at the local high school one evening after work to perform the 1.5-mile run test. She arrives at the track, changes into some exercise clothes, and walks a lap to warm up. The temperature is unseasonably warm (86°F with 75% humidity). Molly begins running and feels pretty good for 200 m; however, she begins to have some difficulty breathing because the pace is too fast for her to maintain. After 600 m Molly starts walking and ends up alternating between running and walking for the rest of the test. Her total test time was 16 minutes. What would be her predicted VO_{2max}? Do you think this is an accurate estimate of her VO_{2max}? What factors, if any, do you think could have contributed to error in the estimation of VO_{2max}? Do you think this was the best choice of a test for Molly? Explain your answer.

REFERENCES

1. Ainsworth BE, Haskell WL, Whitt MC, et al. Compendium of physical activities: an update of activity codes and MET intensities. *Med Sci Sports Exerc*. 2000;32:S498–516.
2. Borg G. *Borg's Perceived Exertion and Pain Scales*. Champaign (IL) 1998: Human Kinetics.
3. Conley DS, Cureton KJ, Dengel DR, Weyand PG. Validation of the 12-min swim as a field test of peak aerobic power in young men. *Med Sci Sports Exerc*. 1991;23:766–73.
4. Davies CT. Limitations to the prediction of maximum oxygen intake from cardiac frequency measurements. *J Appl Physiol*. 1968;24:700–06.
5. Golding LA. *YMCA Fitness Testing and Assessment Manual*. Champaign (IL) 1989: Human Kinetics.
6. Kaminsky LA, Wehrli KW, Mahon AD, Robbins GC, Powers DL, Whaley MH. Evaluation of a shallow water running test for the estimation of peak aerobic power. *Med Sci Sports Exerc*. 1993;25:1287–92.
7. Kilne G, Porcari JP, Hintermeister R, et al. Estimation of VO_{2max} from a one mile track walk, gender, age and body weight. *Med Sci Sports Exerc*. 1987;19:253.
8. Maldonado-Martìn S, Brubaker PH, Kaminsky LA, Moore JB, Stewart KP, Kitzman DW. The relationship of six-minute walk to VO_{2peak} and VT in older heart failure patients. *Med Sci Sports Exerc*. 2006;38:1047–53.
9. McArdle WD, Katch FI, Pechar GS, Jacobson L, Ruck S. Reliability and interrelationships between maximal oxygen uptake, physical work capacity and step test scores in college women. *Med Sci Sports*. 1972;4:182–86.
10. Montoye HJ. The Harvard step test and work capacity. *Rev Can Biol*. 1953;11:491–9.
11. Ryhming I. A nomogram for calculation of aerobic capacity [physical fitness] from pulse rate during submaximal work. *J Appl Physiol*. 1954;7:218–21.
12. Whaley MH, Kaminsky LA, Dwyer GB, Getchell LH, Norton JA. Predictors of over- and underachievement of age-predicted maximal heart rate. *Med Sci Sports Exerc*. 1992;24:1173–79.

Cardiorespiratory Fitness: Maximal Exercise Testing

RISKS

Physical activity and exercise are usually associated with positive health outcomes; however, as was discussed in Chapter 2, there may be some risks associated with exercise. In general, the risks associated with exercise increase both with the intensity of exercise and with an increase in client risk stratification levels. Thus, maximal exercise testing involves a higher degree of risk than the other health-related physical fitness (HRPF) assessments covered previously in this manual.

ACSM's Guidelines for Exercise Testing and Prescription, 8th edition (*GETP8*) provides a review of the risks associated with exercise and exercise testing. Table 8.1 shows a summary of surveys that have been performed to evaluate the cardiovascular risks and complications that have been documented as occurring with maximal exercise testing. The *GETP8* also provides a thorough overview of procedures for maximal exercise tests used in clinical settings. This manual will focus on the use of maximal exercise testing for an HRPF assessment, primarily for low-risk clients.

CONTRAINDICATIONS

The risk stratification procedures covered in Chapter 2 should be reviewed. Particular attention should be given to Box 2.2, which provides the contraindications for exercise testing. It is essential to make sure the screening process employed rules out the presence of any absolute or relative contraindications prior to allowing the client to perform an exercise test.

MONITORING

The primary outcome measure of a health-related cardiorespiratory fitness (CRF) assessment is the measurement of $\dot{V}O_{2max}$. This requires measuring the client's ventilation and the concentrations of O_2 and CO_2 in the inspired and expired air during the maximal exercise test. Although heart rate (HR) is not required to calculate $\dot{V}O_{2max}$, it is typically measured throughout the maximal exercise test. It is also essential to monitor the client for signs and symptoms of exercise intolerance, which would indicate early termination of the test.

Maximal exercise tests are also performed in preventative and rehabilitative exercise program settings and in clinical settings. In these settings, additional monitoring, including exercise electrocardiography, blood pressure, and measurement of O_2 saturation, is standard. The *GETP8* provides a thorough overview of the procedures used in clinical exercise testing settings.

Because the opportunity exists to gather more information during maximal exercise testing, other measures are routinely performed with the assessment of CRF. Table 8.2 provides recommendations for the timing of monitoring measures for maximal exercise testing. These additional monitoring measures require trained staff and some additional equipment, which are common to most clinical exercise facilities. Indications for terminating the test are provided in Box 8.1.

PERSONNEL

The *GETP8* recommends the following:

> In all situations where exercise testing is performed, site personnel should at least be certified at a level of basic life support (CPR) and have automated external defibrillator (AED) training. Preferably, one or more staff members should also be certified in first aid and advanced cardiac life support (ACLS).

TABLE 8.1. CARDIAC COMPLICATIONS DURING EXERCISE TESTING[a]

REFERENCE	YEAR	SITE	NO. TESTS	MI	VF	DEATH	HOSPITALIZATION	COMMENT
Rochmis (12)	1971	73 U.S. centers	170,000	NA	NA	1	3	34% of tests were symptom limited; 50% of deaths in 8 hr; 50% over next 4 days
Irving (5)	1977	15 Seattle facilities	10,700	NA	4.67	0	NR	
McHenry (8)	1977	Hospital	12,000	0	0	0	0	
Atterhog (1)	1979	20 Swedish centers	50,000	0.8	0.8	6.4	5.2	
Stuart (13)	1980	1,375 U.S. centers	518,448	3.58	4.78	0.5	NR	VF includes other dysrhythmias requiring treatment
Gibbons (4)	1989	Cooper Clinic	71,914	0.56	0.29	0	NR	Only 4% of men and 2% of women had CVD
Knight (7)	1995	Geisinger Cardiology Service	28,133	1.42	1.77	0	NR	25% were inpatient tests supervised by non-MDs

MI, myocardial infarction; VF, ventricular fibrillation; CVD, atherosclerotic cardiovascular disease; MD, medical doctor; NA, not applicable; NR, not reported.

[a]Events are per 10,000 tests.

From American College of Sports Medicine. *ACSM's Guidelines for Exercise Testing and Prescription*, 3rd ed. Philadelphia (PA): Wolters Kluwer Health Ltd: 2009, 13 p.

TABLE 8.2. RECOMMENDATIONS FOR THE TIMING OF MONITORING MEASURES

VARIABLE	BEFORE EXERCISE TEST	DURING EXERCISE TEST	AFTER EXERCISE TEST
ECG	Monitored continuously; recorded supine position and posture of exercise	Monitored continuously; recorded during the last 15 s of each stage (interval protocol) or the last 15 s of each 2-min period (ramp protocols)	Monitored continuously; recorded immediately postexercise, during the last 15 s of first min of recovery, and then every 2 min thereafter
HR[b]	Monitored continuously; recorded supine position and posture of exercise	Monitored continuously; recorded during the last 5 s of each min	Monitored continuously; recorded during the last 5 s of each min
BP[a,b]	Measured and recorded in supine position and posture of exercise	Measured and recorded during the last 45 s of each stage (interval protocol) or the last 45 s of each 2-min period (ramp protocols)	Measured and recorded immediately postexercise and then every 2 min thereafter
Signs and symptoms	Monitored continuously; recorded as observed	Monitored continuously; recorded as observed	Monitored continuously; recorded as observed
RPE	Explain scale	Recorded during the last 5 s of each min	Obtain peak exercise value then not measured in recovery
Gas exchange	Baseline reading to assure proper operational status	Measured continuously	Generally not needed in recovery

ECG, electrocardiogram; HR, heart rate; BP, blood pressure; RPE, ratings of perceived exertion.

[a]An unchanged or decreasing systolic blood pressure with increasing workloads should be retaken (i.e., verified immediately).

[b]In addition, BP and HR should be assessed and recorded whenever adverse symptoms or abnormal ECG changes occur.

Reprinted from Brubaker PH, Kaminsky LA, Whaley MH. *Coronary artery disease*. Champaign (IL): Human Kinetics, 2002, 182 p., with permission.

This recommendation points out some facility and equipment requirements for laboratories, specifically access to an AED as shown in Figure 8.1 and first aid equipment. The facility also needs to have a written set of emergency procedures with a regular schedule of drills in which all personnel must participate as illustrated in Figure 8.2.

The guidelines for the recommendations for supervision of testing were presented in Figure 2.2 in Chapter 2 of this manual. The *GETP8* also provides the

BOX 8.1   Indications for Terminating Exercise Testing

ABSOLUTE INDICATIONS

- Drop in systolic blood pressure of >10 mmHg from baseline[a] blood pressure despite an increase in workload when accompanied by other evidence of ischemia
- Moderately severe angina (defined as 3 on standard scale)
- Increasing nervous system symptoms (e.g., ataxia, dizziness, or near syncope)
- Signs of poor perfusion (cyanosis or pallor)
- Technical difficulties monitoring the ECG or systolic blood pressure
- Subject's desire to stop
- Sustained ventricular tachycardia
- ST elevation (+1.0 mm) in leads without diagnostic Q-waves (other than V_1 or aVR)

RELATIVE INDICATIONS

- Drop in systolic blood pressure of >10 mmHg from baseline[a] blood pressure despite an increase in workload in the absence of other evidence of ischemia
- ST or QRS changes such as excessive ST depression (>2 mm horizontal or downsloping ST-segment depression) or marked axis shift
- Arrhythmias other than sustained ventricular tachycardia, including multifocal PVCs, triplets of PVCs, supraventricular tachycardia, heart block, or bradyarrhythmias
- Fatigue, shortness of breath, wheezing, leg cramps, or claudication
- Development of bundle-branch block or intraventricular conduction delay that cannot be distinguished from ventricular tachycardia
- Increasing chest pain
- Hypertensive response (systolic blood pressure of >250 mmHg and/or a diastolic blood pressure of >115 mmHg).

ECG, electrocardiogram; PVC, premature ventricular contraction.

[a]Baseline refers to a measurement obtained immediately before the test and in the same posture as the test is being performed.

Modified from American College of Sports Medicine. *ACSM's Guidelines for Exercise Testing and Prescription,* 8th ed. Philadelphia (PA): Wolters Kluwer Health Ltd: 2009, 119 p.

From Gibbons RJ, Balady GJ, Bricker J, et al. ACC/AHA 2002 guideline update for exercise testing: a report of the American College of Cardiology/American Heart Association Task Force on Practice Guidelines (Committee on Exercise Testing). *Circulation.* 2002;106(14):1883–1892.

following guidance concerning the need for physician supervision of maximal exercise tests:

> The degree of medical supervision of exercise testing varies appropriately from physician supervised tests to situations in which there may be no physician present. The degree of physician supervision may differ with local policies and circumstances, the health status of the patient, and the training and experience of the laboratory staff. Physicians responsible for supervising exercise testing should meet or exceed the minimal competencies for supervision and interpretation of results as established by the AHA.

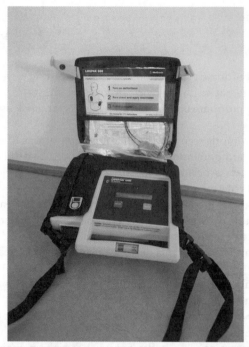

FIGURE 8.1. An automated external defibrillator is essential in all physical fitness assessment settings.

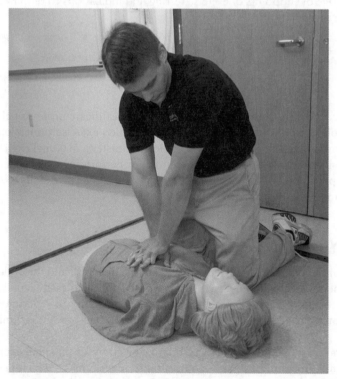

FIGURE 8.2. Regular emergency procedure drills should include a practice session of cardiopulmonary resuscitation (CPR).

BOX 8.2	Cognitive Skills Required to Competently Supervise Exercise Tests

- Knowledge of appropriate indications for exercise testing
- Knowledge of alternative physiologic cardiovascular tests
- Knowledge of appropriate contraindications, risks, and risk assessment of testing
- Knowledge to promptly recognize and treat complications of exercise testing
- Competence in cardiopulmonary resuscitation and successful completion of an American Heart Association–sponsored course in advance cardiovascular life support and renewal on a regular basis
- Knowledge of various exercise protocols and indications for each
- Knowledge of basic cardiovascular and exercise physiology, including hemodynamic response to exercise
- Knowledge of cardiac arrhythmia and the ability to recognize and treat serious arrhythmias
- Knowledge of cardiovascular drugs and how they can affect exercise performance, hemodynamics, and the electrocardiogram
- Knowledge of the effects of age and disease on hemodynamic and the electrocardiographic response to exercise
- Knowledge of principles and details of exercise testing, including proper lead placement and skin preparation
- Knowledge of endpoints of exercise testing and indications to terminate exercise testing

From American College of Sports Medicine. *ACSM's Guidelines for Exercise Testing and Prescription*, 8th ed. Philadelphia (PA): Wolters Kluwer Health Ltd: 2009, 122 p.

Thus, it is accepted that a trained and experienced healthcare professional, such as an American College of Sports Medicine (ACSM)-certified exercise professional with the requisite knowledge, skills, and abilities, could administer a maximal exercise test. The knowledge, skills, and abilities that are required for performing exercise testing are addressed in Appendix D of the *GETP8*. Also, a list of the cognitive skills required of exercise test supervisors is provided in Box 8.2.

SELECTING THE MODE FOR TESTING

The most common modes for exercise testing are the treadmill and the cycle ergometer. These two modes are commonly used because of the ability to easily replicate and control work rates. Arm ergometers, which also have the ability to replicate and control work rates, are utilized for individuals with disabilities that prevent or limit the use of their legs.

For several reasons, the default or standard, selection for maximal exercise testing is the treadmill. Treadmill exercise requires more muscle mass, which generally produces the highest $\dot{V}O_{2max}$. Additionally, there is more experience with use of treadmills for testing in the United States, and for the majority of people, walking is the most common form of daily movement. Unless compelling reasons exist, the choice for exercise mode is typically the treadmill.

The cycle ergometer may be the preferred mode in certain situations. If the client was a trained cyclist or desired to exercise primarily on a cycle ergometer, then a cycle test would be appropriate. The principle of specificity, which was discussed in Chapter 5, applies in this situation. The cycle might also be selected if the client had a disability, injury, or health condition that would make walking difficult or could actually be worsened by walking. Individuals who are obese may be better served by a cycle that helps support body weight (as opposed to the treadmill, in which the individual's body must support all weight). Other reasons for selecting a cycle ergometer may be related to facility issues (such as space and power supply), lower cost, more portability, and quieter operation.

PROTOCOLS

Once the decision on mode of exercise is made, the testing supervisor needs to determine which test protocol to employ. It is wise to set one standard, or default, protocol that will be used most typically within a given facility. A standard protocol allows for both easy assessments of expected responses during the test as well as comparisons between tests. There are appropriate reasons for altering the standard protocol and some principles that should guide this process. One determining factor is whether the protocol will result in a maximal effort between 6 and 15 minutes (ideally between 8 and 12 minutes). A second consideration, applicable only to treadmill tests, is whether the work rate should be increased only through an increase in grade (i.e., a fixed speed protocol) or by increasing both speed and grade. The last consideration is how to increment the work rates, either in stages or as a slow, continuous increase (ramp style).

There are many standardized protocols from which to choose, as indicated in Figure 8.3. Some facilities choose to individualize the protocol to reach a target test time associated with a pretest prediction of the client's $\dot{V}O_{2max}$ based on client characteristics. Typically these individualized protocols are determined by a computer program found on some commercial exercise testing systems. It is beyond the scope of this manual to provide a thorough explanation of many different protocols including arm ergometer protocols; however, the most commonly used protocols that would be applicable to HRPF assessment are reviewed. These include the most frequently used clinical protocol (Bruce), a fixed-speed walking protocol (Balke), a standardized treadmill ramping protocol (Ball State University [BSU]/Bruce), a treadmill running protocol (Costill/Fox), and a cycle protocol.

BRUCE PROTOCOL

Dr. Robert Bruce, a cardiologist, developed the Bruce protocol, which has been used in clinical exercise testing laboratories for approximately 40 years (3). Surveys of exercise testing laboratories in the United States have consistently reported the Bruce protocol, or modified versions, to be the one most (82%) commonly used (9). This popularity is in part a result of the substantial amount of data on the typical responses expected with the Bruce protocol, including predictions of $\dot{V}O_{2max}$, based on treadmill time, as will be reviewed later in this chapter.

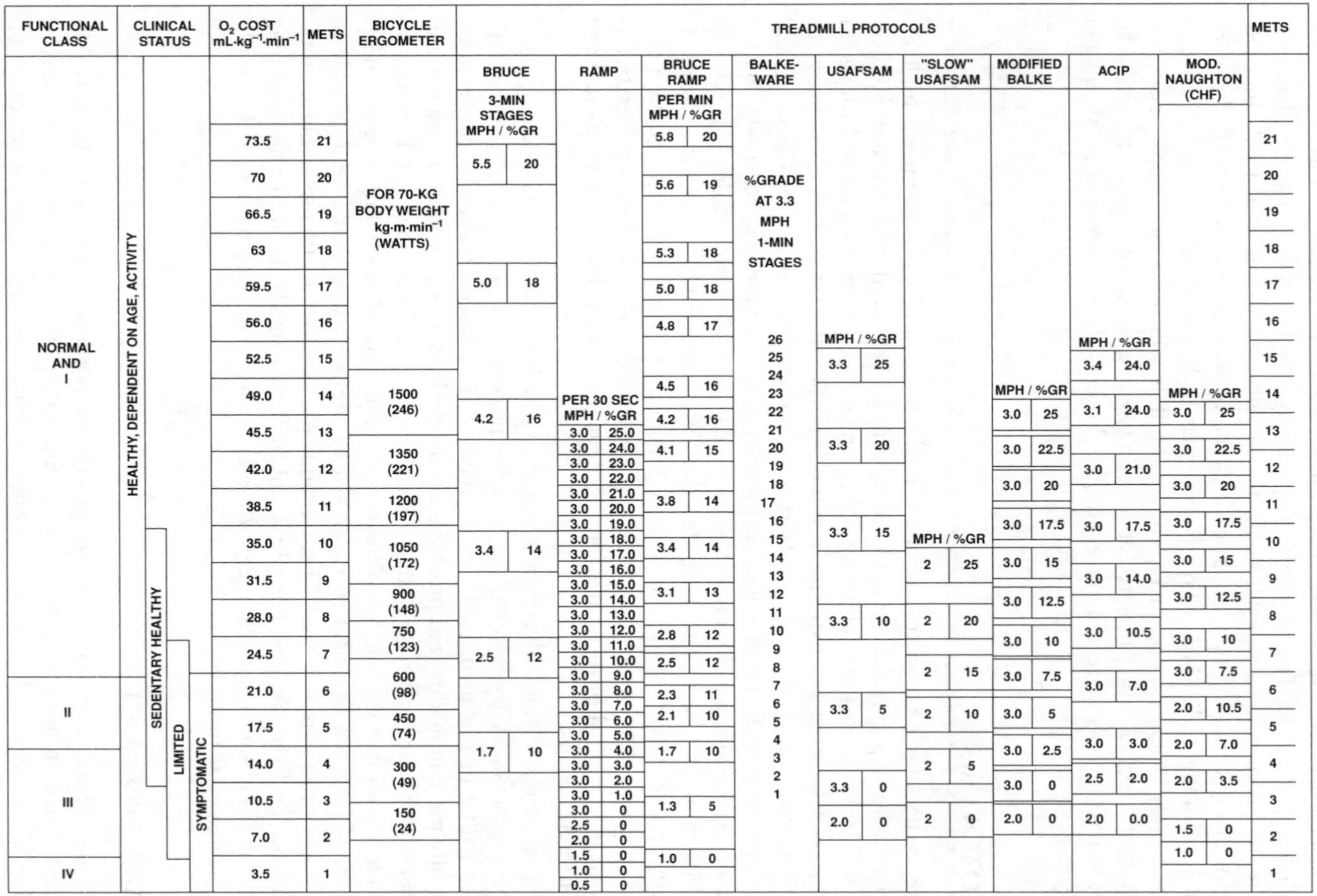

FIGURE 8.3. Common exercise protocols and associated metabolic costs of each stage. Adapted from American College of Sports Medicine. *ACSM's Guidelines for Exercise Testing and Prescription*, 8th ed. Philadelphia (PA): Wolters Kluwer Health Ltd: 2009, 114–115 p.

Functional class / Clinical status (left margin):

- FUNCTIONAL CLASS: NORMAL AND I (top, highest METS) · II · III · IV (lowest METS)
- CLINICAL STATUS: HEALTHY, DEPENDENT ON AGE, ACTIVITY (top span) · SEDENTARY HEALTHY · LIMITED · SYMPTOMATIC (lowest)

Metabolic costs and protocols (values shown as MPH / %GR unless noted):

METS	O₂ COST (mL·kg⁻¹·min⁻¹)	BICYCLE ERGOMETER kg·m·min⁻¹ (WATTS), 70-kg	BRUCE 3-MIN STAGES	BRUCE RAMP (per min)	BALKE-WARE (%GRADE @ 3.3 MPH, 1-min stages)	USAFSAM	"SLOW" USAFSAM	MODIFIED BALKE	ACIP	MOD. NAUGHTON (CHF)
21	73.5			5.8/20						
20	70									
19	66.5			5.6/19						
18	63		5.5/20	5.3/18						
17	59.5			5.0/18						
16	56.0		5.0/18	4.8/17						
15	52.5					3.3/25			3.4/24.0	
14	49.0	1500 (246)		4.5/16	26			3.0/25	3.1/24.0	3.0/25
13	45.5	1350 (221)	4.2/16	4.2/16 · 4.1/15	22			3.0/22.5		3.0/22.5
12	42.0	1200 (197)		3.8/14	20	3.3/20		3.0/20	3.0/21.0	3.0/20
11	38.5				17					
10	35.0	1050 (172)	3.4/14	3.4/14	15	3.3/15	2/25	3.0/17.5	3.0/17.5	3.0/17.5
9	31.5	900 (148)		3.1/13	12			3.0/15	3.0/14.0	3.0/15
8	28.0	750 (123)		2.8/12	10	3.3/10	2/20	3.0/12.5	3.0/10.5	3.0/12.5
7	24.5		2.5/12	2.5/12	8			3.0/10		3.0/10
6	21.0	600 (98)		2.3/11 · 2.1/10	6	3.3/5	2/15	3.0/7.5	3.0/7.0	3.0/7.5
5	17.5	450 (74)	1.7/10	1.7/10	3		2/10	3.0/5	3.0/3.0	2.0/10.5
4	14.0	300 (49)			1	3.3/0	2/5	3.0/2.5	2.5/2.0	2.0/7.0
3	10.5	150 (24)		1.3/5		2.0/0		3.0/0	2.0/0.0	2.0/3.5
2	7.0			1.0/0			2/0	2.0/0		1.5/0
1	3.5									1.0/0

RAMP protocol (per 30 sec, 3.0 MPH, %GR): grade decreases in 1% steps — 3.0/25.0, 3.0/24.0, 3.0/23.0, 3.0/22.0, 3.0/21.0, 3.0/20.0, 3.0/19.0, 3.0/18.0, 3.0/17.0, 3.0/16.0, 3.0/15.0, 3.0/14.0, 3.0/13.0, 3.0/12.0, 3.0/11.0, 3.0/10.0, 3.0/9.0, 3.0/8.0, 3.0/7.0, 3.0/6.0, 3.0/5.0, 3.0/4.0, 3.0/3.0, 3.0/2.0, 3.0/1.0, then 2.5/0, 2.0/0, 1.5/0, 1.0/0, 0.5/0.

TABLE 8.3. BRUCE TREADMILL PROTOCOL (3)

STAGE	TIME (min:sec)	SPEED (mph)	GRADE (%)
1	0:00	1.7	10.0
2	3:00	2.5	12.0
3	6:00	3.4	14.0
4	9:00	4.2	18.0
5	12:00	5.0	18.0
6	15:00	5.5	20.0
7	18:00	6.0	22.0

Note: a modification for less fit clients is to add one or two preliminary stages:

STAGE	TIME (min:sec)	SPEED (mph)	GRADE (%)
0	0:00	1.7	0.0
0.5	3:00	2.5	5.0

See Figure 8.3 for estimated metabolic equivalent levels.

From Bruce RA, Hosmer F, Kusumi F. Maximal oxygen intake and nomographic assessment of functional aerobic impairment in cardiovascular disease. *Am Heart J.* 1973;85:546–62.

The Bruce protocol consists of 3-minute stages, where the speed and grade both increase with each stage, and the work rate increment is approximately 3 metabolic equivalents (METs) per stage. The initial stage of this protocol is set at a MET level of 4.6, which may be too large of a requirement for deconditioned adults, many elderly individuals, and cardiac and pulmonary patients. A modified version of this protocol includes either one or two preliminary stages (stages 0 and 0.5) as shown in Table 8.3.

BALKE-WARE PROTOCOL

Another commonly used treadmill protocol is the Balke-Ware, developed by Dr. Bruno Balke and colleagues (2). The main features of this protocol are that it is of fixed speed and the rate of increment in work rate is relatively small ($\approx$0.5 METs) at each stage (1 minute). There have been several modifications made to this protocol, one of which has been employed routinely over the years at the Cooper Clinic in Dallas, Texas, and that has produced the normative chart for interpreting CRF. The original Balke-Ware protocol and some common modifications are shown in Table 8.4.

BALL STATE UNIVERSITY/BRUCE RAMP PROTOCOL

Ramp protocols increase the workload more gradually, usually by shortening the stage time and decreasing the work rate increments. Although ramp protocols for cycle ergometers have been available for a longer period of time, systems to provide ramping increments for treadmills have only been available since the 1990s. Owing to the well-known features of the Bruce protocol, a standardized ramping variation of this protocol was developed. The BSU/Bruce ramp protocol increases the work rate every 20 seconds ($\approx$1 MET/minute) and has speed and grade settings identical to the Bruce protocol at every 3-minute period during the test (6). This test protocol is displayed

TABLE 8.4. ORIGINAL AND MODIFICATIONS OF THE BALKE-WARE TREADMILL PROTOCOL (2)

	ORIGINAL					MODIFIED[a]		
STAGE	TIME (min:sec)	SPEED (mph)	GRADE (%)		STAGE	TIME (min:sec)	SPEED (mph)	GRADE (%)
1	0:00	3.3	1.0		1	0:00	3.0	0.0
2	1:00	3.3	2.0		2	2:00	3.0	2.5
3	2:00	3.3	3.0		3	4:00	3.0	5.0
4	3:00	3.3	4.0		4	6:00	3.0	7.5
5	4:00	3.3	5.0		5	8:00	3.0	10.0
6	5:00	3.3	6.0		6	10:00	3.0	12.5
7	6:00	3.3	7.0		7	12:00	3.0	15.0
8	7:00	3.3	8.0		8	14:00	3.0	17.5
9	8:00	3.3	9.0		9	16:00	3.0	20.0
10	9:00	3.3	10.0		10	18:00	3.0	22.5
11	10:00	3.3	11.0		11	20:00	3.0	25.0
13	12:00	3.3	13.0					
14	13:00	3.3	14.0					
15	14:00	3.3	15.0					
16	15:00	3.3	16.0					
17	16:00	3.3	17.0					
18	17:00	3.3	18.0					
19	18:00	3.3	19.0					
20	19:00	3.3	20.0					
21	20:00	3.3	21.0					
22	21:00	3.3	22.0					
23	22:00	3.3	23.0					
24	23:00	3.3	24.0					
25	24:00	3.3	25.0					
26	25:00	3.3	26.0					

[a]The speed for the modified protocol can be selected to meet the comfort level of the patient. Other common variations are 2.0 and 2.5 mph. See Figure 8.3 for estimated metabolic equivalent levels.

From Balke B, Ware R. An experimental study of physical fitness of Air Force personnel. *U S Armed Forces Med J.* 1959;10:675.

within Table 8.5. Monitoring intervals are typically the same as for the standard Bruce protocol. One beneficial feature of this protocol is the ability of the client to walk for a longer period of time than during the standard Bruce protocol. Clients typically have to start running as they begin stage 4 of the Bruce protocol (minute 9), compared to minute 11 of the BSU/Bruce protocol.

RUNNING PROTOCOL

As the principle of specificity would suggest, trained endurance runners will perform best on a protocol that allows them to run at faster speeds and lower elevations than the treadmill tests described above. Obviously, running protocols will limit the ability to obtain and monitor variables like blood pressure and heart function, with the use of an electrocardiogram, during the exercise test. Thus, these types of protocols are only indicated for low-risk individuals who regularly train for endurance by running. The protocols typically feature a beginning phase where the client runs at a moderate pace for a couple of minutes to warm up followed by a rapid increase to the peak sustained running speed desired by the client. Further increments in work are obtained by making

TABLE 8.5. **THE BALL STATE UNIVERSITY (BSU)/BRUCE TREADMILL RAMP PROTOCOL (6)**

STAGE	TIME (min:sec)	SPEED (mph)	GRADE (%)	STAGE	TIME (min:sec)	SPEED (mph)	GRADE (%)
1	0:00	1.7	0.0	33	10:40	4.0	15.2
2	0:20	1.7	1.3	34	11:00	4.1	15.4
3	0:40	1.7	2.5	35	11:20	4.2	15.6
4	1:00	1.7	3.7	36	11:40	4.2	16.0
5	1:20	1.7	5.0	37	12:00	4.3	16.2
6	1:40	1.7	6.2	38	12:20	4.4	16.4
7	2:00	1.7	7.5	39	12:40	4.5	16.6
8	2:20	1.7	8.7	40	13:00	4.6	16.8
9	2:40	1.7	10.0	41	13:20	4.7	17.0
10	3:00	1.8	10.2	42	13:40	4.8	17.2
11	3:20	1.9	10.2	43	14:00	4.9	17.4
12	3:40	2.0	10.5	44	14:20	5.0	17.6
13	4:00	2.1	10.7	45	14:40	5.0	18.0
14	4:20	2.2	10.9	46	15:00	5.1	18.0
15	4:40	2.3	11.2	47	15:20	5.1	18.5
16	5:00	2.4	11.2	48	15:40	5.2	18.5
17	5:20	2.5	11.6	49	16:00	5.2	19.0
18	5:40	2.5	12.0	50	16:20	5.3	19.0
19	6:00	2.6	12.2	51	16:40	5.3	19.5
20	6:20	2.7	12.4	52	17:00	5.4	19.5
21	6:40	2.8	12.7	53	17:20	5.4	20.0
22	7:00	2.9	12.9	54	17:40	5.5	20.0
23	7:20	3.0	13.1	55	18:00	5.6	20.0
24	7:40	3.1	13.4	56	18:20	5.6	20.5
25	8:00	3.2	13.6	57	18:40	5.7	20.5
26	8:20	3.3	13.8	58	19:00	5.7	21.0
27	8:40	3.4	14.0	59	19:20	5.8	21.0
28	9:00	3.5	14.2	60	19:40	5.8	21.5
29	9:20	3.6	14.4	61	20:00	5.9	21.5
30	9:40	3.7	14.6	62	20:20	5.9	22.0
31	10:00	3.8	14.8	63	20:40	6.0	22.0
32	10:20	3.9	15.0				

From Kaminsky LA, Whaley MH. Evaluation of a new standardized ramp protocol: the BSU/Bruce Ramp protocol. *J Cardiopulm Rehabil.* 1998;18:438–44.

modest increases in grade until the client reaches maximum capacity. A modified Costill/Fox protocol is shown in Table 8.6 (14).

CYCLE PROTOCOLS

The most unique factor in selecting a cycling protocol is that because it is a non–weight-bearing mode of exercise, the workload is set by pedaling against an external resistance. The ability to push this resistance will be determined to a large degree by the amount of muscle mass a person possesses. Although the absolute level of work will be greater for the larger person, CRF is measured in units relative to body weight (i.e., $mL \cdot kg^{-1} \cdot min^{-1}$). Table 8.7 shows one commonly used protocol for cycle testing, which uses 2-minute stages with work rate increments of $150 \ kg \cdot m \cdot min^{-1}$. When testing a larger person, the protocol may start with a higher workload or it may use larger increments during the test.

Ramp protocols are quite popular for cycle ergometry testing. As noted earlier, commercial exercise testing systems will commonly provide a program to develop the ramping protocols.

TABLE 8.6. MODIFIED COSTILL/FOX RUNNING PROTOCOL (14)

STAGE	TIME (min)	SPEED (km · h^{-1})	GRADE (%)
Warm-up	0–4	5.0	0.0
Speed increasing stages[a]	4 each	9.5	0.0
		12.0	
		13.5	
		16.0	
Grade increasing stages	2 each		2.0
			4.0
			6.0
			8.0

[a]Speed continues to increase until the subject reports an RPE of 13. At that point the speed remains constant and the grade increases by 2% every 2 min until exhaustion.

From Trappe SW, Costill DL, Vukovich MD, Jones J, Melham T. Aging among elite distance runners: a 22-yr longitudinal study. *J Appl Physiol.* 1996;80:285–90.

TEST PROCEDURES

Multiple personnel are needed to administer maximal exercise testing, with the exact number being determined by the amount of monitoring used. A list of the primary job responsibilities is provided below, with modifications made to reduce the number of staff if less monitoring is performed or if the staff are very experienced and can perform multiple responsibilities during a test.

SUPERVISOR

This person acting as test supervisor will have performed a pretest review of the client's risk stratification screening information, making sure there are no contraindications for testing. The informed consent document is reviewed again (note: this would have already been completed at the risk stratification screening) and the exercise test procedures are outlined. The supervisor should make sure the client understands that although the objective is to work to a maximal effort level, the test can be stopped at any time and the staff should be promptly informed if anything unusual is experienced during the test (particularly symptoms of ischemia such as chest discomfort). An explanation of the rating of perceived exertion (RPE) scale should be provided at this time. The supervisor may also perform one of the test technician roles during the test.

TABLE 8.7. AN EXAMPLE OF A CYCLE TEST PROTOCOL

STAGE	TIME (min:sec)	WORK RATE (kg · m · min^{-1})
1	0:00	300
2	3:00	600
3	6:00	900
4	9:00	1,200
5	12:00	1,500
6	15:00	1,800
7	18:00	2,100

Note: For smaller individuals and women, the work rates may need to be reduced by 50%; for heavier individuals and/or well-trained cyclists, the duration of each stage can be reduced to 2 minutes.

TEST MONITORING ROLES

The most commonly monitored variables during the test are the electrocardiogram or other measure of HR, metabolic measurements, blood pressure (BP), perceived exertion, and possibly oxygen saturation. Additionally, the treadmill or cycle ergometer work rates need to be controlled by the staff, or monitored by the staff if controlled by a computer program.

The protocol should start with a brief 1- to 2-minute warm-up (treadmill—slow speed of walking; cycle—unloaded pedaling). During this time the staff should be making sure all equipment is functioning properly and the client is relatively comfortable on the exercise ergometer. When the staff and the client are ready, the protocol begins and the sequence of measures as described in Table 8.2 is performed. To ensure client safety, it is important that all staff observe the client during the test and that one specific staff member is assigned this responsibility as a primary role. In many laboratories, the technician performing the BP measurements will also obtain measures of RPE and become the primary observer and communicator with the client. One staff member is typically in charge of recording data (HR, BP, RPE, symptoms) during the test. The technician monitoring the electrocardiogram, or other monitor of HR, commonly performs this duty. Also, one technician monitors the readings from the metabolic measurements and can control the workload changes during the test. This technician would also be responsible for the pretest calibration of the metabolic cart and the posttest cleaning and sterilization of the mouthpiece and breathing valve used by the client. The staff should provide feedback to the client throughout the test and encourage a maximal effort. Common objective indicators of maximal effort are a respiratory exchange ratio of ≥ 1.1, a plateau in $\dot{V}O_2$ (no further increase in $\dot{V}O_2$ with an increase in work rate), and achievement of age-predicted maximal HR. Subjective indicators include an RPE of 18, 19, or 20 and the client's appearance of exhaustion.

MEASURED AND ESTIMATED $\dot{V}O_{2max}$

To provide the gold standard measure of CRF, the maximal exercise test must include the assessment of $\dot{V}O_2$ with a metabolic measurement system. These systems will provide measures of exercise ventilation and expired concentrations of O_2 and CO_2 to derive the measurement of $\dot{V}O_2$. These metabolic measurement systems can also provide a detailed recording of the responses throughout the test and can be used to provide other data of interest to the client (e.g., ventilatory threshold).

The measurement of $\dot{V}O_2$ is not always feasible, as metabolic measurement systems are relatively expensive to purchase and to maintain. These systems also require additional expertise of the personnel operating them and interpreting results. Fortunately, there are methods to predict $\dot{V}O_{2max}$ from measurements obtained during a maximal exercise test.

ESTIMATING $\dot{V}O_{2max}$ FROM EXERCISE TEST TIME

Several research reports have provided regression equations to obtain an estimate of $\dot{V}O_{2max}$ from exercise test duration. When using prediction models, it is critical that the identical protocol be followed for the test, and that the subjects are not allowed to use handrail support during the treadmill test. It is also important to know the general characteristics of the population that was assessed in the study. Box 8.3 provides prediction

BOX 8.3	Prediction of $\dot{V}O_{2max}$ from Treadmill Test Time

BRUCE PROTOCOL

Healthy persons (3)

$$\dot{V}O_{2max} (mL \cdot kg^{-1} \cdot min^{-1}) = 6.7 - 2.82 \text{ (men} = 1, \text{women} = 2)$$
$$+ 0.056 \text{ (time in sec)}$$

Healthy men and women (n = 296)

$$\dot{V}O_{2max} (mL \cdot kg^{-1} \cdot min^{-1}) = 3.814 \text{ (time in min)} - 3.938 \pm 4.68 \quad (r = 0.87)$$

(Unpublished data—Ball State University [BSU] Adult Physical Fitness Program)

BSU-BRUCE RAMP PROTOCOL (6)

Men and women (n = 392)

$$\dot{V}O_{2max} (mL \cdot kg^{-1} \cdot min^{-1}) = 3.9 \text{ (time in min)} - 7.0 \pm 3.4 \quad (r = 0.93)$$

BALKE PROTOCOL

Women (n = 49)—3.0 mph protocol with 2.5%/3 min (11)

$$\dot{V}O_{2max} (mL \cdot kg^{-1} \cdot min^{-1}) = 0.023 \text{ (time in sec)} + 5.2 \pm 2.7 \quad (r = 0.94)$$

Men (n = 51)—3.3 mph protocol (10)

$$\dot{V}O_{2max} (mL \cdot kg^{-1} \cdot min^{-1}) = 1.444 \text{ (time in min)} + 14.99 \pm 0.025 \quad (r = 0.92)$$

equations for the Bruce, BSU/Bruce ramp, and Balke-Ware protocols. The reference tables for CRF interpretation (Tables 7.3 and 7.4) also provide an estimate for the modified Balke protocol used at the Cooper Clinic.

ESTIMATING $\dot{V}O_{2max}$ FROM PEAK WORKLOAD

Another approach to obtaining an estimate of $\dot{V}O_{2max}$ is to use the ACSM metabolic calculations. This method is not desirable as the metabolic calculation equations were developed for steady-state submaximal work rates. However, for cycle testing or other treadmill protocols without prediction equations based on test time, they are sometimes used.

INTERPRETATION

As with other measures of HRPF, no national standard has been developed and accepted for interpreting CRF. However, the ACSM has long used the data developed by the Cooper Clinic in Dallas, Texas, as a source for providing interpretations of CRF assessments. These CRF gender-specific charts were provided in Tables 7.3 and 7.4. Similar to the body composition norms, it is important to recognize that these values are based on the population that has received these measures and are expressed as percentiles, which may limit their usefulness for interpreting test results from populations with different characteristics.

SUMMARY

The gold standard measure of CRF is the maximal exercise test with measurement of ventilation and the concentrations of O_2 and CO_2 in the inspired and expired air. Because of the increased risks for the client to perform this test, the relatively expensive equipment required to obtain the necessary measurements, and the high level of training required of the testing personnel, this procedure is not routinely performed in all HRPF assessment settings. However, fitness professionals working in preventative and rehabilitative exercise programs will often be involved in performing this form of assessment of CRF.

> > > LABORATORY ACTIVITIES

MAXIMAL EXERCISE TESTS

Data Collection
Our class will perform three maximal exercise tests, one each on three different subjects. One student will perform a BSU/Bruce treadmill protocol, one student will perform a modified Costill/Fox running protocol, and one student will perform a maximal test on a cycle ergometer. Follow the instructions for monitoring and test administration presented in this chapter. For each test, a different group of students will perform the roles of the different technicians.

Laboratory Report
1. Using the exercise test data recording sheet (p. 164), make a graph for each test of the HR (x-axis) and $\dot{V}O_2$ (y-axis) relationship.
2. Did all subjects reach a true $\dot{V}O_{2max}$? What objective criteria indicate they did or did not give a maximal effort? Interpret the test results for each subject.
3. For the cycle test, pretend we stopped the test after the subject completed two stages with HR values between 110 and 150 bpm. Use those submaximal data to predict $\dot{V}O_{2max}$ using the methods discussed in Chapter 7. How does this predicted value compare to the measured value from the maximal exercise test?
4. Use the prediction formula based on treadmill test time for the BSU/Bruce ramp test to predict $\dot{V}O_{2max}$. How does this predicted value compare to the measured value from the maximal exercise test?
5. Which submaximal assessment (performed by these subjects in the labs from Chapter 7) predicted actual $\dot{V}O_{2max}$ the best for each subject? Discuss why this particular submaximal test may have been a better predictor than the other tests for that subject.

> > > CASE STUDY

Marge is a 42-year-old sedentary woman who came to the ABC Fitness Club to have her cardiorespiratory fitness measured. She chose to have a maximal exercise test done to measure her $\dot{V}O_{2max}$. The testing supervisor selected the standard Bruce protocol for the test and Marge completed 6 minutes and 42 seconds before she signaled that she needed to stop the exercise test. Her measured maximal HR was 183 bpm and she rated her RPE as 19. Unfortunately, there were technical problems with the metabolic cart and no data were available. Can you provide a prediction of Marge's $\dot{V}O_{2max}$ based on the exercise test data? If so, how would you interpret the $\dot{V}O_{2max}$? Do you agree that this was the best protocol for Marge? If so, explain why. If not, which protocol would you have selected and why would you have selected this alternate protocol?

REFERENCES

1. Atterhog JH, Jonsson B, Samuelsson R. Exercise testing: a prospective study of complication rates. *Am Heart J.* 1979;98:572–79.
2. Balke B, Ware R. An experimental study of physical fitness of Air Force personnel. *U S Armed Forces Med J.* 1959;10:675.
3. Bruce RA, Hosmer F, Kusumi F. Maximal oxygen intake and nomographic assessment of functional aerobic impairment in cardiovascular disease. *Am Heart J.* 1973;85:546–62.
4. Gibbons L, Blair SN, Kohl HW, Cooper K. The safety of maximal exercise testing. *Circulation.* 1989;80: 846–52.
5. Irving JB, Bruce RA, DeRouen TA. Variations in and significance of systolic pressure during maximal exercise (treadmill) testing. *Am J Cardiol.* 1977;39:841–48.
6. Kaminsky LA, Whaley MH. Evaluation of a new standardized ramp protocol: the BSU/Bruce Ramp protocol. *J Cardiopulm Rehabil.* 1998;18:438–44.
7. Knight JA, Laubach CA Jr, Butcher RJ, Menapace FJ. Supervision of clinical exercise testing by exercise physiologists. *Am J Cardiol.* 1995;75(5):390–91.
8. McHenry PL. Risks of graded exercise testing. *Am J Cardiol.* 1977;39(6):935–37.
9. Myers JN, Voodi L, Froelicher VF. A survey of exercise testing: methods, utilization, interpretation, and safety in the VAHCS. *Med Sci Sports Exerc.* 2000;32:S143.
10. Pollock ML, Bohannon RL, Cooper KH, Ayers J, Ward A, White S, Linnerud A. A comparative analysis of four protocols for maximal treadmill stress testing. *Am Heart J.* 1976;92:39–46.
11. Pollock ML, Foster C, Schmidt D, Hellman C, Linnerud AC, Ward A. Comparative analysis of physiologic responses to three different maximal graded exercise test protocols in healthy women. *Am Heart J.* 1982; 103:363–73.
12. Rochmis P, Blackburn H. Exercise tests. A survey of procedures, safety, and litigation experience in approximately 170,000 tests. *JAMA.* 1971;217(8):1061–66.
13. Stuart RJ, Ellestad MH. National survey of exercise stress testing facilities. *Chest.* 1980;77(1):94–7.
14. Trappe SW, Costill DL, Vukovich MD, Jones J, Melham T. Aging among elite distance runners: a 22-yr longitudinal study. *J Appl Physiol.* 1996;80:285–90.

Conversions

LENGTH/HEIGHT

1 kilometer = 1,000 meters (m)
1 kilometer = 0.62137 miles
1 mile = 1,609.35 meters
1 meter = 100 centimeters = 1,000 millimeters (mm)
1 foot = 0.3048 meters
1 meter = 3.281 feet = 39.37 inches
1 inch = 2.54 centimeters (cm)
0.394 inches = 1 centimeter

MASS OR WEIGHT

1 kilogram = 1,000 grams = 10 Newtons (N)
1 kilogram = 2.2 pounds
1 pound = 0.454 kilograms
1 gram = 1,000 milligrams (mg)
1 pound = 453.592 grams (g)
1 ounce = 28.3495 grams
1 gram = 0.035 ounces

VOLUME

1 liter = 1,000 milliliters (ml)
1 liter = 1.05 quarts
1 quart = 0.9464 liters
1 milliliter = 1 cubic centimeter (cc or cm^3)
1 gallon = 3.785 liters (L)

WORK

1 Newton-meter = 1 Joule (J)
1 Newton-meter = 0.7375 foot-pounds
1 foot-pound = 1.36 Newton-meters
1 kiloJoule (1,000 J) = 0.234 kilocalories (kcal)

1 foot-pound = 0.1383 kilograms per meter (kg · m)
1 kg · m = 7.23 foot-pounds

VELOCITY

1 meter per second (m · sec^{-1}) = 2.2372 miles per hour (mph)
1 mile per hour = 26.8 meters per minute (m · min^{-1}) = 1.6093 kilometers per hour (kph)

POWER

1 kilogram-meter per minute (kg · m^{-1} · min^{-1}) = 0.1635 watts (W)
1 watt = 6.12 kg · m^{-1} · min^{-1}
1 kg · m^{-1} · min^{-1} = 1 kp · m^{-1} · min^{-1}
1 watt = 1 Joule per second (J · sec^{-1})
1 horsepower (hp) = 745.7 watts

TEMPERATURE

1 degree Celsius = 1 degree Kelvin = 1.8 degrees Fahrenheit
1 degree Fahrenheit = 0.56 degrees Celsius

METRIC ROOTS

deci = 1/10
centi = 1/100
milli = 1/1,000
kilo = 1,000

Forms[1]

Risk Stratification Assessment
Body Composition Data Form
Muscular Fitness Data Form
Flexibility Data Form
Submaximal Cycle Test Data Form
Exercise Test Data Form

---

[1]All forms used with the permission of the Ball State University Clinical Exercise Physiology Program

RISK STRATIFICATION ASSESSMENT

NAME: _____ Test Date: _____ AGE: _____GENDER (circle one) M F

Age	Yes No		
Family History	Yes No	If yes, who/what _____	
Cigarette Smoker	Yes No		
Hypertension	Yes No	Resting BP _____ mmHg	Medication Yes No

Hypercholes-   Yes No LDL _____ mg $\cdot$ dL^{-1} HDL _____ mg $\cdot$ dL^{-1} Medication   Yes No
  terolemia

Impaired Fasting Yes No FG _____ mg $\cdot$ dL^{-1} Medication   Yes No
  Glucose

Obesity   Yes No BMI _____ kg $\cdot$ m^{-2} Waist _____ cm

Physical Inactivity Yes No Vig. PA 20 min/3 days Yes No Mod. PA 30 min/5days   Yes No

High HDL   Yes No

Signs or symptoms of cardiovascular/pulmonary disease (check all that apply):

____ chest discomfort   ____ paroxysmal noc. dyspnea   ____ ankle edema

____ shortness of breath   ____ known heart murmur   ____ syncope   ___ none

____ intermittent claudication   ____ palpitations/tachycardia   ____ unusual fatigue

MEDICAL HISTORY

Cardiac: Yes No   If yes, explain _____

Pulmonary: Yes No   If yes, explain _____

Metabolic: Yes No   If yes, explain _____

List Medications: _____

_____

_____

_____

Risk Stratification (circle one):	**Low Risk**	**Moderate Risk**	**High Risk**

_____   _____

Testing Staff Name   Date

See Table 2.2 for Risk Factor Thresholds
See Table 2.3 for Symptoms of Cardiovascular, Pulmonary, or Metabolic Diseases
See Table 2.1 for Risk Stratification Criteria

BODY COMPOSITION DATA FORM

_____   _____   _____   _____
Client Name   Date   Technician(s)   File #

Weight History Review

Weight at age 18_____lbs
  Cyclic Wt Loss? <u>Y/N</u>
Recent Wt Loss? <u>Y/N</u> if yes (lbs, time)_____
Previous Body Comp. Data (% fat, wt, date)_____

Visual Impression Record

%fat appearance: (circle one)
  <10 10–15 15–20 20–25 25–30 >30
Overall appearance:
  Lean / Muscular / Average / Fat

Body Comp Considerations:

_____   Exercise (last 3 hrs): <u>Y/N</u>   Eating (last 3 hrs): <u>Y/N</u>   Void (last 1 hr): <u>Y/N</u>

Height / Weight   Weight (nearest 0.25 lb) _____lb / 2.2046 = _____kg
Height (nearest 0.25 in) _____in × 0.0254 = _____m
Body Mass Index (kg $\cdot$ m^{-2}) _____kg / (_____ m × _____m) = _____

Circumferences (cm)

	1	2	3	Mean
Waist	____	____	____	____
Hip	____	____	____	____

Waist Hip Ratio: _____

Skinfolds (mm)

Sex	Site	1	2	3	Mean
W	Triceps	____	____	____	____
W	Suprailiac	____	____	____	____
W	Thigh	____	____	____	____
	alternate	____	____	____	____
M	Chest	____	____	____	____
M	Abdomen	____	____	____	____
M	Thigh	____	____	____	____

*Body Density: 1._ _ _

*%Fat (3 site): _____

Staff Comments:_____
_____
_____

*See below: **3- Site Formula** and *Conversion of Body Density (Db) to Percent Body Fat*

3-Site Skinfold Formulas by gender:

Men: Body Density = 1.112 − 0.00043499 (SSF__) + 0.00000055 (SSF__)^2 − 0.00028826 (Age__)

Women: Body Density = 1.097 −0.00046971 (SSF__) + 0.00000056 (SSF__)^2 − 0.00012828 (Age__)

Body Density (Db) to Percent Body Fat Conversion by age/ gender:

Men ages 20- 80yrs.: (4.95/Db) − 4.50

Women ages 20- 80yrs.: (5.01/Db) − 4.57

Staff Comments: _____

MUSCULAR FITNESS DATA FORM

_____   _____   _____   _____
Client Name   Date   Technician(s)   ID #

Age: _____ Gender: ____Weight: _____ lb _____ kg Height: _____ in _____ cm

Strength Assessment

Right Hand Grip Strength
Trial 1 (kg)   Trial 2 (kg)   Trial 3 (kg)   **Best Score (kg)**
_____   _____   _____   _____

Left Hand Grip Strength
Trial 1 (kg)   Trial 2 (kg)   Trial 3 (kg)   **Best Score (kg)**
_____   _____   _____   _____

Combined Score: _____   Classification: _____

1 – RM Bench Press Strength
Trial 1 (kg)   Trial 2 (kg)   Trial 3 (kg)   **Best Score (kg)**   **Ratio**
_____   _____   _____   _____   _____

Classification: _____

1 – RM Leg Press Strength
Trial 1 (kg)   Trial 2 (kg)   Trial 3 (kg)   **Best Score (kg)**   **Ratio**
_____   _____   _____   _____   _____

Classification: _____

Endurance Assessment

YMCA Submaximal Bench Press
Total Number of Lifts _____

Classification: _____

Push-Up Test
Total Number of Push-ups _____
Classification: _____

Curl-Up Test
Total Number of Curl-ups _____

Classification: _____

FLEXIBILITY DATA FORM

_____   _____   _____   _____
Client Name   Date   Technician(s)   ID #

Age: _____ Gender: ____Weight: _____ lb _____ kg Height: _____ in _____ cm

Sit and Reach Test
Trial 1 (in)   Trial 2 (in)   Trial 3 (in)   **Best Score (in)**
_____   _____   _____   _____

'Zero'Point: _____ Inches____   Classification: _____

Sit and Reach Test
Trial 1 (cm)   Trial 2 (cm)   Trial 3 (cm)   **Best Score (cm)**
_____   _____   _____   _____

'Zero'Point: _____ cm_____   Classification: _____

Lumbar Extension Test
Trial 1 (in)   Trial 2 (in)   Trial 3 (in)   **Best Score (in)**
_____   _____   _____   _____

Classification: _____

Lumbar Flexion Test
Trial 1 (in)   Trial 2 (in)   Trial 3 (in)   **Best Score (in)**
_____   _____   _____   _____

Classification: _____
Range of Motion Assessments.

Flexibility Test	Measured Range of Motion
Shoulder Flexion	
Shoulder Extension	
Shoulder Internal Rotation	
Shoulder External Rotation	
Hip Flexion (testing leg fully extended)	
Hip Flexion (testing knee flexed 90° and hip flexed 90°)	
Hip Extension (testing leg fully extended)	
Hip Abduction	
Hip Adduction	

SUBMAXIMAL CYCLE TEST DATA FORM

Name: _____ Age: _____ Sex: _____ Date: _____

Time of test: _____ ID #:_____

Rest HR: _____ Rest BP:_____
           supine / sitting   supine / sitting

Weight: _____ lb _____ kg Height: _____ in _____ cm

RISK STRATIFICATION:_____

Hours since last meal? _____ List food and/or beverages: _____

MEDICATIONS: Dose   Time last taken
_____

_____

_____

ACTIVITY/EXERCISE HISTORY: _____

PAST ET: Date: _____ HR_{max}: _____ BP_{max}: ___/___ VO_{2max}: _____ Test Time: ____ Protocol: _____

Minute	Resistance (kg)	$kg \cdot m \cdot min^{-1}$	Pulse Palpation (15 sec)	HR Monitor (bpm)	BP (mm Hg)	RPE
1						
2						
3						
4						
5						
6						
7						
8						
9						
10						
11						
12						
Recovery 1						
Recovery 2						
Recovery 3						

Estimated VO_{2max}: _____

Fitness Classification: _____

EXERCISE TEST DATA FORM

Name: _____ Age: _____ Sex: _____ Date: _____

Time of test: _____ ID #: _____

Rest HR: _____ Rest BP: _____
           supine / sitting*   supine / sitting*

Weight: _____ lb _____ kg Height: _____ in _____ cm

RISK STRATIFICATION: _____

Hours since last meal? _____   List food and/or beverages: _____

MEDICATIONS: Dose   Time last taken

_____

_____

_____

ACTIVITY/EXERCISE HISTORY: _____

PAST ET: Date: _____ HR_{max}: _____ BP_{max}: ___/___ VO_{2max}: _____ Test Time: ____ Protocol: _____

Protocol: _____

Time (min)	Work setting	HR (bpm)	BP (mm HG)	RPE	Comments
0–1	/		/		
1–2	/		/		
2–3	/		/		
3–4	/		/		
4–5	/		/		
5–6	/		/		
6–7	/		/		
7–8	/		/		
8–9	/		/		
9–10	/		/		
10–11	/		/		
11–12	/		/		
12–13	/		/		
13–14	/		/		
14–15	/		/		

Immediate Post-Test Symptoms:	Chest Discomfort	SOB	Lightheadedness	Other	
RECOVERY					**ACTIVE or SUPINE**
0–1			/		
1–2			/		
2–3			/		
3–4			/		
4–5			/		

REASON for STOPPING TEST: _____

TECH 1:_____   TECH 2: _____   SUPERVISOR: _____

_____

Note: work setting is speed and grade for the treadmill or resistance and rpms for the cycle.
* Use standing for a treadmill test.

Index

Note: Page numbers followed by b, f, or t indicate boxed, figures, or table material.